Praise for **For the Love of Beef**

"Scott Lively has given us a fascinating peek into the hidden world of American beef. This book is not only chock-full of need-to-know facts—from humane handling to nutritional differences—but it is also an entertaining read you won't want to put down. *For the Love of Beef* hits the bull's-eye!"

DR. MARK HYMAN, founder and director,
The UltraWellness Center; *New York Times*–bestselling author

"Whether you're an expert beef industry insider or a casual consumer, you'll find *For the Love of Beef* compelling, informative and entertaining. Bravo!"

LARRY PERKINS, president and COO, Perkins Food Service

"Who would have thought a book about beef would be a page-turner and fun to read? But that is certainly the case with Scott Lively's *For the Love of Beef*. It's full of fascinating tidbits and written in an entertaining, irreverent style that makes you both laugh and cringe. I loved it."

ROBIN COOK, *New York Times*–bestselling author

"*For the Love of Beef* covers a very complex topic in an easy-to-follow and entertaining fashion. For beef lovers and non-beef lovers alike, this book gives a great view into the beef industry and allows the reader to walk away with a better understanding."

MATT WALTERS, director, meat procurement, H-E-B Grocery Company

"Scott Lively handles critical data with ease. *For the Love of Beef* is a valuable resource for anyone interested in smart food choices. Scott fearlessly exposes the reality for American beef consumers. An entertaining and resourceful piece to share with your best food friends!"

MARK KING, owner, 2 Sustain; former chairman,
USDA National Organic Standards Board

FOR THE
LOVE
OF BEEF

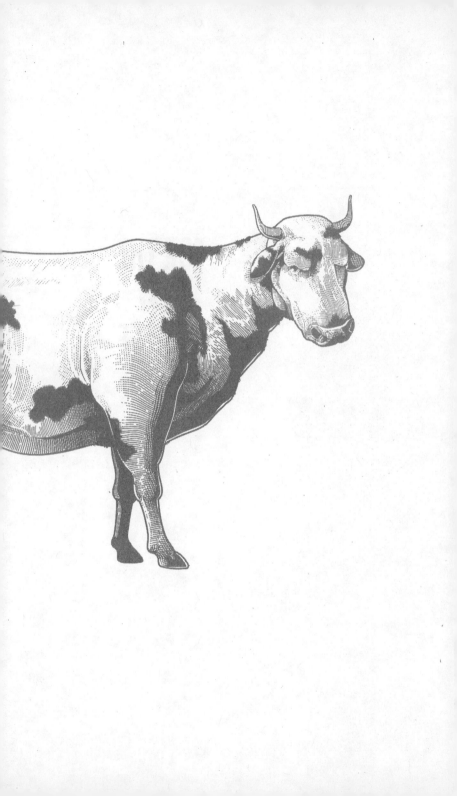

SCOTT LIVELY

FOR THE LOVE OF BEEF

The Good, the Bad and the Future of America's Favorite Meat

PAGE TWO

Cataloguing in publication information is
available from Library and Archives Canada.
ISBN 978-1-77458-002-8 (paperback)
ISBN 978-1-77458-114-8 (ebook)

Page Two
pagetwo.com

Writing/research services by Patti McCracken
Edited by James Harbeck
Copyedited by Jenny Govier
Proofread by Alison Strobel

Cover and interior design by Peter Cocking
Cover photo by igorr1/iStock
Interior illustrations by Michelle Clement
Frontispiece by man-Half-tube/iStock

Printed and bound in Canada by Friesens
Distributed in Canada by Raincoast Books
Distributed in the US and
internationally by Macmillan

21 22 23 24 25   5 4 3 2 1

fortheloveofbeef.com

Contents

Introduction

_____

BACK IN the 1940s, the Big Beef folks had a spectacularly bad idea. It was such a colossally bad idea they put into play that the cattle industry was crippled by it for about a decade afterward.

They had taken their cue from the new suburbia, where cookie-cutter homes were springing up, built for the cookie-cutter families that had been spit out after World War II as if they'd come off an assembly line: trim white father, petite white mother and their two white children, who were all now living in a tidy little house in a row of tidy little houses.

The so-called American family had drastically shrunk, but more to the point, there was now an icebox in every tidy little kitchen, where a small amount of beef could be stored for the small white family. Perfect, said Beef. We'll give them small cows.

For as long as there had been a cattle industry in America, ranchers had liked to produce big, fat cows. The more, the better, they'd always figured. More cow meant more tallow to make more candles and soap, more bone to make more fertilizer, and more meat for, well, more meat.

But America had changed, and the Big Beef guys wanted a made-to-order smaller cow for the made-to-order smaller families. A cookie-cutter cow. A cow that could literally fit into a box. Boxed beef was what they were after.

The breed they ended up with looked like a B-movie beast. The cows were short, pot-bellied, pug-nosed dwarfs. They had sad, crooked legs. They snorted when they breathed. It was like a pig had made love to a dog and this was the offspring. And the poor Frankenmeat animals were not at all healthy.

But Big Beef was doing what it had always done, and what it absolutely still does today: striving to make itself indispensable to you. And as a $111 billion-a-year industry, it's pretty good at it, despite the occasional mistakes.

You can now stock in that "icebox"—which has gotten far bigger than your grandparents' 1940s icebox—all manner of cuts: chuck, shank, rib, sirloin, you name it. Your steak can be a tomahawk with five more inches of extra rib bone. It can be marbled, or not; it can be bone-in, or not. It can be Angus or Hereford, or Wagyu, or grass-fed, or corn-fed, or organic. There is more on tap for the American beef eater than there has ever been. It's enough to make you swoon.

The beef industry is giving you everything it knows how to give you and telling you everything it wants you to know, while revealing very little.

How do I know this? Well, I am part of Big Beef. I've been in the commercial beef business for more than fifteen years.

When I was thirty-two years old, I abandoned a successful career in IT to buy an old, out-of-use meat packing facility in Howard, South Dakota, near where my then-wife hailed from. At the time, I knew nothing about the beef industry. However, my wife was obsessed with health, wellness and organic foods, and that drove me. I went out and bought thirty head of cattle in Seward, Illinois, had them processed at a local packing house, and sold the meat door-to-door to Chicago restaurants out of the back of a Volvo wagon. The business took off from there. I started it because I wanted to bring back a dying town and truly promote rural economic development. Instead, I created what became one of the largest organic beef companies in America, Dakota Beef.

Today I am the president of Raise American, a company I co-founded. Raise American is now the largest producer of sustainable, organic, grass-fed beef in the nation.

Beef is to the American palate what sunshine is to beaches, what popcorn is to movies, what a hot dog is to a ballpark. Beef is not about something to eat, it's an anthem to eating. The average American eats around fifty-seven pounds of beef a year. (Surprisingly, only 5 percent of Americans are vegetarian. Even fewer Americans are vegan.) We eat hamburger, ribeye, meatballs. We eat beef in tacos, lasagna, casseroles and pizza toppings. We have found there is no end to how we can use beef to trick out any recipe we decide to put to the test. We enjoy beef as a main course, a side dish, a stuffing, a seasoning.

We don't eat beef to stay alive, we eat it to *feel* alive. There are any number of ways to get the good stuff it gives us—the

B vitamins, the protein. Just ask a vegetarian, many of whom are probably "flexitarians" anyway because they can't say no to a delicious hamburger. Rather, we eat beef for the experience. We eat it for the texture, the aroma, the atmosphere. Whether it be prepared in a backyard or a bistro, beef is as good as our birthright. Look at it this way: the French have their wine, the Germans have their beer and the Americans have their beef.

Yet, what do we really know about our beef and where it comes from? How well do we know the big steaks on our plates or the ground beef in our freezers? Where is it from? Is it from Texas, Nebraska, Uruguay or Australia? Is it true that the meat from thousands of cows is in just one pound of hamburger? How is that possible, and how safe is it? What about hormones and antibiotics? Is Certified Angus Beef really from Angus cattle, and how do we verify this?

Is Kobe beef really Kobe beef? And what makes Kobe beef so special? Is my US beef really from the USA, or did it come from South America? (And why am I not being told?) Does fat always add flavor? What does "prime rib" even mean? Why am I being sold meat that's "on the bone"? How lean is lean? In whose world is a three-inch steak better than a half-inch steak? And what's in my hamburger?

What is good fat and what is bad fat? What am I paying extra for what I don't need?

And what is flap meat?

We love beef, but we don't know beef.

Everything I know about the beef industry, I learned from the ground up. I'm like the kid who starts out sweeping floors at the local grocer and grows up to become the owner of a chain of grocery stores. I know every cut of beef as if I cut it myself. I know the weight of it in my hand like a pitcher knows a baseball. I can tell you how it's washed and how it's wrapped. I can tell you how it's aged and how it's stored. I can tell you how many hands have been on it and how many miles it's traveled. I can tell you the precise dimensions of the truck that transports it. I love beef and I know beef. It's time you knew it, too.

I want you to know what the waiter doesn't. I want you to know what the butcher doesn't. I want you to know what the packers and grocers and the government know but don't have to tell you. I want you to know it's not always what you think it is. I want you to know the truth.

If a sommelier brought you a bottle of wine with no label or date on it and said, "We promise you this is superb. It's absolutely worth the $210 you're paying for it," you'd be skeptical. Yet, you might be totally content to spend $50 to $75 for a steak, just based on what the menu says or what the waiter claims it is.

I want you to know what you're eating. I want you to be fearless in asking questions: What is it? Where does it come from? Can I see the label?

I also want you to eat what you want to eat, and not what somebody tells you that you should eat. Each person's relationship with beef is personal—as personal as wine, chocolate or how you like your coffee. When you think of beef, you might think of fine dining: a filet mignon in a cozy, low-lit French restaurant. When I think of beef, I might think to wipe its ass, lop off its horns and burn its hair off. But you like what you like, and I like what I like. And no one should tell either one of us otherwise. Not the waiter (who is reading from a script), not the butcher (who is often just a meat handler there to stock the shelves), not what's trending on the Food Network. And certainly not just what fits in "the box." It should be about you. What you want.

And you should be well enough informed, and experienced enough, to truly know what you do and don't enjoy.

A recent study conducted for the meat industry by a company called 210 Analytics showed that younger consumers are particularly interested in knowing about their beef: where it came from and how it was sourced. I believe every beef eater, and certainly every beef lover, should have easy, ready-made access to that information, and far more.

I want to arm you with this information and I want you to know for yourself, "This is probably not Prime Angus; this is probably a low 'Choice' product." I want you to see yellow fat and know what that means. My goal is for beef eaters like you to be able to look at a cut of beef and tell the difference between what is clean, green and healthy and what came from old dairy cow (or "cull," as the cows are called when they get too old to produce milk). I want you to be able to tell the difference and *taste* the difference.

So think of this book as a handbook for *your* beef: what it is, where it comes from and why it matters. *For the Love of Beef* is a "take-with" reference guide and an eye-opening primer. Just like wine lovers need a field guide to wine, beef lovers need a field guide to beef. I hope you will learn what you need. I hope you will learn what you're not being told but what you *should* be told. I hope you will learn how to ask the right questions of the right people to get the right beef for you and your family.

Most important, I hope you will learn what you *truly* like, not what you're *told* to like.

Take it from me, the beef geek.

PARTS OF THE COW

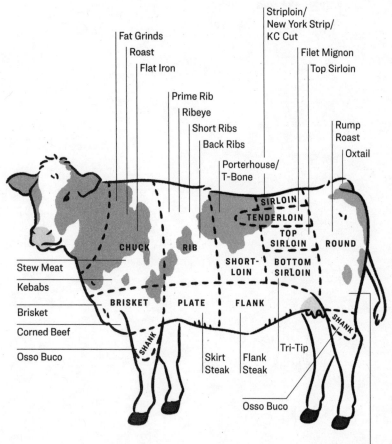

1

So What Is Organic, Anyway?

ARMERS HAVE been farming organically ever since the invention of land and the invention of animals and the invention of farmers. It's just that it used to be called "farming." We didn't need "organic," because "organic farming" would have been as redundant as "wet rain."

But farms became mechanized. Tractors replaced mules. Threshers replaced flails. Then combines replaced threshers. Farmers began to work more land and feed more people. Yet, the more land they worked, the more removed they became from that land—that's the irony life gives us.

They became cogs in a big machine, then a bigger machine, and a bigger machine still, until the process of farming was so industrialized that it seemed perfectly ordinary to put toxic chemicals on crops. It seemed perfectly ordinary to keep chickens cooped up in cages. It seemed perfectly ordinary to cram twelve thousand cows onto a feedlot and shove food at them while they ate it standing in their own shit. Wait, the animals get sick from this? Well, we've got antibiotics for that.

I was out of the country for a bit, and when I came back, I went to the grocery store. From the parking lot, I could see a huge banner across the front doors advertising "antibiotic-free chicken." I'd seen it a hundred times before and it had never caught my eye, but I *didn't* see it abroad, so when I came home it hit me like a punch in the face. Antibiotic-free chicken? Is this what we've come to? That's a selling point? That's the best marketing idea they can come up with? That chicken isn't blasted full of harmful antibiotics? What's next? Will I see a big sign saying, "These plums haven't been dipped in piss"?

Let's take a look at the chemicals. The herbicides that get sprayed on our food and the food the livestock eat were originally engineered by the US Army during World War II. Before then, no one had much experience with pouring man-made chemicals on plants. But whether or not it was trying to, the army discovered a chemical combination that made a good weed killer. Soon, it worked out a more potent weed killer, and by the time the Vietnam War rolled around, military brass figured it would be great as chemical warfare, and they weren't wrong. Agent Orange was sprayed on forests and vegetation to kill the hiding spots of the Viet Cong. But the weed killer was also used to decimate the crops, because doing that could decimate the health of the people for generations to come, the health of the environment and the health of the economy. And it did. Eventually, the army's war-grade weed killer was morphed into a suburban weed killer, which we were told we could use in our yards and on our factory farms. It wasn't war-grade material, but it was hardly safe. It was as if someone said, "Here, let's take this less potent bomb and spray it far and wide on our food supply."

Why organic?

Organic is really just an organized attempt to bring our food quality back to what we had pre-chemicals, pre-antibiotics, pre–caged and crowded, pre-GMO, pre–added hormones. This can't fully be achieved because our soil, air and water are already pretty corrupted. And just because Farmer Sue is growing a field of organic beets doesn't mean the chemicals from Farmer Jasmine's conventional farm won't waft over and invade Sue's beets. But we do what we can.

For decades, farmers have been farming organically without the label. But ever since the government defined the standard in 1990 with the Organic Foods Production Act, this method of farming has permitted farmers to put a USDA seal on their product. It allows them to say, "Look, I followed a certain recognized protocol." The seal has become the most identifiable alternative to conventional beef. The USDA Organic seal has actually become a brand in itself.

To qualify as 100 percent certified organic, specific conditions have to be met. As far as livestock are concerned, the animal must be raised under conditions that provide it access to outdoors, exercise and freedom to roam, although this is negotiable to some degree. Feed has to be grown without herbicides, pesticides, GMOs, animal-derived proteins, added hormones or antibiotics. A farmer or rancher can administer antibiotics if an animal is sick, but that animal must be removed from the herd and can no longer be part of organic production.

The meat itself is processed under strict standards regarding what it can be cleaned with and what chemicals can be used. One of the things most commonly used in this industry is peracetic acid, or even high-quality apple cider vinegar. Most people would be surprised to learn that Bragg apple cider vinegar is used to wash the carcass once the hide is removed. It's also used to clean a lot of the equipment that's used in the processing of the meat. I've always wondered if Bragg even knows that their product is one of the most intensively used cleaning solutions in organic animal beef processing.

There are other standards to be met, too, including how the waste is managed. It must be safely composted. Also, the environment has to be free from sewage and waste-runoff water. In the organic method of farming, tremendous efforts are made, and great expense is taken, to keep the animals and their environment clean and green.

What about grass-fed?

Most certified organic animals are raised on large farms, similar to conventional ones. Organic beef cattle might be "finished"—that means what they eat the last few months before slaughter—at some of the largest feedlots in the country, and some of them are still going to be finished on corn with very little grass. Yes. It's true: some organic cattle are finished on corn. The corn they eat has to be certified organic corn, but still. The truth is, organic cattle are not currently required to be on grass. A lot of people don't know that because the Big Beef guys don't want it to be known. They want beef eaters to assume that organic automatically means grass-fed. It doesn't.

Consumers complain because grass-fed costs more. However, it has a higher price tag because it costs more to raise grass-fed cattle. Those of us in organic grass-fed, we don't have the cheats. We don't shove wagons full of corn down the cow's gullet the last few months, then wash that down with antibiotics while we stick a needle full of hormones in them. We respect the cowiness of the cow. There, I said it. But we do. We let the cows be cows. We let them graze. We let them get to the weight on their own. And that costs more.

I really believe that organic, grass-fed beef—beef that's raised right—is for everybody. I think it belongs in the best restaurants, in high school cafeterias and on food trucks. I think it belongs in our tacos. I think it belongs on our grills. I think it can be everywhere that conventional beef is now.

The rise of organic in this country is historic. For the first time in the life of Big Beef, the consumer is leading market change. Previously, Big Beef was used to driving the market. They brought out a product and told consumers to like it, and consumers did. *Try these new steak tips. Choose "Prime"—it's the best. Angus is the way to go.* That was all Big Beef talking. Decade after decade, it was Big Beef telling beef eaters what to like. But organic is changing that.

Do you really think the beef industry wants to go to the trouble of getting organic beef on your table? Hell, no. It's much cheaper and much easier for the beef guys to stick with conventional. But beef eaters are demanding healthy beef, and Big Beef has finally decided to listen.

2

Why Your Beef Ain't COOL

Y OUR BEEF ain't COOL.

Why do I say that? I'm referring to the Country of Origin Labeling law, which was finalized in Congress in May 2009 and requires labeling that shows which country your food comes from. However, a 2016 spending bill quietly removed beef and pork from the list. COOL regulations are still in place for nearly every other conceivable food: chicken, lamb, goat, farm-raised fish, wild-caught fish, shellfish, pecans, macadamia nuts, ginseng. But not for beef.

Think about it. The government wants you to know where your ginseng comes from, but not your beef.

You should be shocked to know that most of the foreign beef comes from as far away as South America and Australia. The cattle are grown and slaughtered there, then shipped to either the East Coast or the West Coast of the United States.

The beef usually winds up in the Midwest, where it's processed by the big packers.

How much beef is imported is important to know. Let's start with the organic sector. Nearly 80 percent of the organic beef you buy is imported. That's because most organic beef is grass-fed, and the United States imports a lot of grass-fed beef because it's cheaper and more efficient to do so. Grass-fed cattle need green pastures all year long. Kansas can't give them grass year-round. South Dakota sure can't. Texas can, but not in the numbers needed, so the beef guys turn to places like Australia and Uruguay and Argentina. There, grassland is cheap and there's plenty of it, which means the costs all around are lower. This is just too good of a bargain for the packers to pass up. And the packers and grocers know it's important to keep the prices low, because Americans are cheap when it comes to food. Americans pay less for food than any other developed nation.

The market share for organic is growing, but it is still a fraction of the beef that's consumed in this country. So what about the conventional beef, the non-organic supply? That makes up the overwhelming majority of beef that's sold. Most of that beef is from cattle raised in the United States, but not all of it. Up to 15 percent of conventional beef is sourced from other countries.

Fifteen percent may seem like a relatively small slice, but consider that it's a slice of a very, very big pie. It means nearly four billion pounds of beef are imported every year. According to *Inc.* magazine, McDonald's sells one billion pounds of hamburger every year in America. Let me frame it this way:

the amount of beef we import annually equals the amount of beef McDonald's sells in four years.

Now, there's no reason to believe that imported beef isn't, ounce for ounce, on par with American beef as far as food safety and quality goes. In fact, USDA inspectors are all over the world to ensure just that. The issue with COOL isn't that the United States imports beef, it's that you're not required to know it. And not only can packers omit that information (and they do), but beef is allowed to be sold with a label on the package that reads "Product of the USA," even when it very clearly is not.

Well-known, iconic brands buy significant amounts of foreign beef, and the grocery stores they sell it to pass it off as American. They can do this. It's perfectly legal. The law states that as long as the meat was *processed* in America—which is just another way of saying it was put through a grinder in the United States—it can be called an American beef product.

I think you deserve to know whether your beef came from Kansas or whether it came from Uruguay. And if it says "Product of the USA," it should truly be a product of America. It's only fair.

Why was beef removed from the COOL list? One reason was because the big packers wanted it removed. They argued that the record-keeping necessary to comply with COOL was costing them too much. They also complained that COOL was a violation of their freedom of speech. It's hard to figure out when "freedom of speech" turned into "omit and mislead," but the World Trade Organization somehow agreed with the big packers, and before you could say, "Where's the beef (from)?" Congress had removed the COOL chains that Big Beef claimed had been placed around its neck.

Meanwhile, the small packers do *not* import, so as soon as there was no longer a Country of Origin Labeling requirement for beef, the value of their cattle dropped dramatically. These small packers desperately want COOL regulations back, because being able to demonstrate that their product is truly American is a significant advantage.

There are four big meat packers in the United States—JBS, Tyson, Cargill and National Beef—and these Big Four are to the beef industry what Microsoft and Apple are to computers. They control more than 80 percent of the market, wielding mind-blowing influence not only over Congress, but over commerce itself.

So much influence, in fact, that there is a legend within the industry that eighteen-wheelers in this country were specifically built to beef specifications. The semitrucks hold twenty pallets, two thousand pounds each, and those pallets fit within an inch of the cargo space of every standard long-haul truck in America. Regardless of whether it's true that the Big Four designed our big trucks, the fact that the story exists speaks to the power of Big Beef.

But it wasn't always this way. Back in the 1970s, there were four big meat packers, yes, but they had only 20 percent of the market. This left most of the market share in the hands, and from the lands, of local farmers. It was the massive expansion of McDonald's that changed the beef landscape in America.

In its early days, McDonald's bought from more than a hundred suppliers. But as it got bigger and bigger, the burger chain consolidated its operation and eventually only wanted to buy from large meat packers that could scale up their operations. Grocery store chains saw what was happening and stepped in line to do the same thing. The end result was the cattle equivalent of Walmart squashing Main Street.

Big Beef's influence got as big as it did because it was able to rise to the occasion. My hat's off to it for that. But it had a cozy relationship with the Department of Agriculture long before it scaled up for McDonald's. The partnership goes back as far as World War II, and I think cozy is too cozy when the two agree to omit information as to which country your beef comes from.

Is Your Patty Safe?

EFORE WE hit the panic button, it's important to know that the meat you eat undergoes a very rigorous quality control process. And none more than hamburger. The USDA truly does a great job of keeping us safe, no question. Nearly half the meat we consume in this country is ground beef. It is as American as a cold beer on a hot day, and there's not a meal we could sit down to that couldn't be made better with a dash of our holy Holstein mixed in like a blessing. But ground beef isn't just the patty sitting on the bun; it is also in our taco, our meatloaf, our lasagna, our casserole, our spaghetti sauce, our omelet, our stir-fry. It's even sprinkled on our pizza as a topping. And it's in hot dogs!

We. Heart. Ground. Beef.

The burger meat usually comes from older dairy cows, or culls, who are no longer producing milk the way they used to. When these cows are slaughtered, their meat gets turned into ground beef. But you can also get ground beef from "trimmings." There are at least twenty-nine different cuts of beef that can be carved from a side of beef. Meat is trimmed off those cuts, and the leftover parts, the trimmings, are put into cardboard containers that can hold two thousand pounds of beef trimmings. These two-thousand-pound containers could have meat from American, Argentinian, Uruguayan, Australian and Canadian cattle, and each container gets dumped into a giant commercial grinder and turned into ground beef.

This means your one-pound package of ground beef is not meat from one cow. It's meat from thousands of cows. You won't know where it comes from because there's no COOL sticker on it, and you certainly won't know how many cows it came from, but if you think of an auditorium packed with cattle and imagine that DNA from each one of those cows is in your one-pound package of ground beef, you start to get an idea.

Now that you're thinking about all that DNA, let's turn to bacteria.

E. coli is *everywhere. E. coli* is on your phone, your steering wheel, your door handles. It's on your computer, your TV and your kitchen counter. It's even on your floor, your walls and your windows. It's definitely in your yogurt, your butter and your beef. We live with it every day, co-exist with it, without ever knowing it's there, because it's usually only present in trace amounts. But even when there is more than a trace— say, on the surface of your steak—that steak still presents very little food-borne risk to you. Not so with your hamburger.

Here's why. When cattle are slaughtered, the carcasses are washed with high-pressure jets spewing hot water, and these jets wash away any feces, which is where *E. coli* hangs out.

(*E. coli* O157:H7 is the strain associated with beef.) Later, when the meat is cut into steaks, any traces left on the surface will stay on the surface, because *E. coli* cannot penetrate muscle.

So if I pull out a ribeye and slap it on the grill—and I don't do anything to it: I don't wash it or salt it, I just drop it on the grill and cook it for sixty seconds on each side—I've killed all the rest of the bacteria on that meat. If there was *E. coli* on it when I put it on the grill, there's no *E. coli* on it when I've pulled it off, because the bacteria can only be on the surface of the steak, and I burned that off.

But *E. coli* gets into ground beef in ways it can't get into steak, which makes it a far greater danger for infecting you. If even an infinitesimal amount of *E. coli* is present on meat that's about to get ground, a disaster is looming. The *E. coli* is no longer on the surface, but all mixed up in the middle. Kevin Smith, assistant vice president and general manager of Costco Wholesale Corporation in Tracy, California, has probably seen more beef ground into hamburger than anyone else on Earth, and he explains it this way: "If you had a giant glass bowl full of white marbles and there was just one black marble in the bowl, you could reach your hand in there all day and never grasp the black marble." But if I took that bowl and I ground it, really pulverized it, and mixed all that fine powder up, I could scoop it with my spoon and have a little bit of black marble in every spoonful. *That* is *E. coli* in hamburger.

So why aren't our hamburgers making us sick? For one thing, packing houses today have become very efficient and very mechanized, which means less human intervention than ever before. Fewer humans means fewer hands on the beef. Adding to that, hamburger meat is often being packed in retail-ready trays by a machine at the packing house—another mechanized step that keeps hands away. Fewer hands means far less chance of bacterial contamination. The notion of the neighborhood butcher is quaint, but the butcher handles your beef far more than your average grocery store does, which can increase your risk. The fewer hands, the better.

And the USDA has a strong system in place to keep our beef safe. They learned their lesson back in 1993, when four children died and 750 people fell ill after eating hamburgers from Jack in the Box that were contaminated with a deadly strain of *E. coli*. Up to that point, the best method the USDA could come up with for testing beef was the old "poke and sniff," which is as self-evident as it is disturbing. Inspectors would touch the carcass, then smell it to determine if it was "off"—the same way someone might sniff a carton of milk.

The Jack in the Box tragedy awoke the USDA to its shortcomings, and before long a rigorous system was set up called Hazard Analysis and Critical Control Point, known as HACCP, which all packing houses across America are now required to maintain. It calls for microbial testing to detect the presence of harmful bacteria, such as *E. coli*.

Inspectors also examine the animals coming into the slaughterhouse, and the carcasses are examined again after the animals have been killed. The inspectors also make sure the meat is being kept at correct temperatures and that the facilities are clean and sanitary.

Incidentally, there is something in the beef industry called "*E. coli* positive trimmings"—or they used to be called that.

Now they're called "presumptive positive." These are trimmings that *could* contain *E. coli* because a plate count test showed a high degree of bacteria. Instead of being thrown out, these trimmings are categorized as "FCO"—For Cooked Only—and used in pre-cooked meat that's sold in frozen dinners, or in frozen meatballs, or in any kind of pre-cooked meats available in the freezer section of the grocery store. There is virtually no risk to the consumer here. The *E. coli* is definitely cooked out of the meat. As an absolute OCD freak and self-described beef snob, I would have no problem eating a further processed item that I knew came from an FCO meat product, because I know the science behind it and I'm comfortable with it.

Ground beef, in any case, should always be cooked to an internal temperature of 160°F to absolutely ensure that any food-borne bacteria that might still be lurking is killed off. Some people use a food thermometer, which is the safest way to check if your meat is fully cooked.

E. coli is a pathogen, and pathogens are hard to control, but the USDA has done a great job of keeping the American beef supply clean and healthy. The beef industry couldn't feed millions of people and kill nearly a hundred thousand animals a day and have the level of healthy food in this country that it does without the high standard set by the USDA.

4

What's Prime and Who Decides?

T HE "KING OF MEATS"—the prime rib—is so revered in this country that it was finally given a whole day devoted to its indulgence. April 27th is National Prime Rib Day, a day to tuck your checkered napkin under your chin, grab your fork and knife and praise gluttony.

This particular cut of beef is called prime rib because it comes from the primal section of ribs on the cow, ribs six through twelve. But if "prime" is printed anywhere on your menu other than right next to "rib," then the beef being served up better be USDA Prime, which is a different kind of prime altogether. Prime rib is a cut of beef, whereas USDA Prime is a grade the government gives beef.

The USDA has eight grades it gives meat, and the top three are Prime, Choice and Select. This is not a grade for quality, but a grade for flavor, or what the USDA thinks flavor should look like. And to the USDA, flavor means fat.

Does the USDA look at the outer layer of fat? No, not that fat. What the USDA deems valuable is the intramuscular fat, or IMF, a network of tiny fat vessels laced through the meat. The IMF has no membrane, or has one so thin it is easily penetrated, and this is the fat that gives your meat more flavor. The more IMF in a cut of beef, the more marbled it will look, and the most marbled of all gets a USDA Prime label.

This way of appraising beef in America goes back more than a hundred years, when Professor Herbert Mumford decided there should be some kind of grading system. Mumford was head of the Department of Animal Husbandry at University of Illinois, and he took his cue from the public school grading system that had just come into place. He set forth a series of criteria, which included descriptions and photographs of what he classified as seven grades of meat, the first three of which were named Prime, Choice and Good.

Within about fifteen years, Mumford's grading system led the government to adopt his general system, and eventually, the grading of agricultural products was authorized in 1946 when Congress passed the Agricultural Marketing Act.

As far as the average beef eater is concerned, little has changed since Mumford first devised his grading system in 1902. "Good" was eventually changed to "Select" in 1987, and somewhere along the way an eighth category was squeezed in, but that's about it. Grading is voluntary. If a packer wants their beef graded, they pay the USDA to come out and grade it.

But who really decides what's Prime and what's not? Turns out, it's a man with a card with a picture of beef on it. Not much has changed since Mumford's day, because that's more or less how it was done back in 1902, too.

The beef grader has a card with pictures of steak on it, each labeled Prime, Choice or Select and each steak showing varying amounts of marbling. The grader takes a look at the chilled carcass about a day after slaughter. He (the graders are still largely male) looks at the ribeye carcass between the twelfth and thirteenth ribs, and compares it to the card he's holding in his hand. With that, he judges what category the meat falls into (mostly Select, Choice or Prime). That's it. He eyeballs it based on an image. That's how the USDA measures the quality of your beef. Which is like saying, "This house was built with bricks; therefore, it must be the very best house," without bothering to factor in the house's age, its size, the neighborhood the house is in, how well the house has been cared for or even the construction firm that built it. Or whether you even like brick.

There are so many factors that can contribute to, or detract from, the flavor of your beef that it's nearly pointless to measure only one factor, and especially pointless to employ the USDA to do it, given you can look at a frozen cut of meat yourself and see how much marbling is present.

And really, who is to say what tastes good? The USDA? Taste is for you to decide. You might really like a grass-fed filet mignon, and I might like a well-marbled, good old-fashioned Angus ribeye. And both of us are right to like what we like. No one should be able to tell you, "This is the best steak."

The USDA is going to continue to send graders into the packing houses to judge what's Prime and what's not, but honestly, there's no better tool than your own palate for measuring taste.

HOW BEEF MAKES THE GRADE

The beef grading system originated more than a hundred years ago, and really took hold after World War II, when Congress passed the Agricultural Marketing Act in 1946. It was a way to imply quality and therefore increase demand for corn-fed cattle, which began to be heavily produced then.

Grading is not mandatory. Beef producers volunteer to have their meat graded. The grade determination is based on the amount of marbling in the beef, or intramuscular fat (IMF), a distinctive feature of corn-fed cattle. Grass-fed or organic beef is rarely graded.

Who is a grader?

A grader is an inspector who is certified and employed by the USDA. The inspector does not need to have any particular background or expertise and usually gets their training on the job.

Where is the grading done?

The graders inspect the carcass right at the facility where the cattle are harvested. They are only interested in one very specific area of the carcass, and that is the ribeye between the twelfth and thirteenth ribs. Based on what the graders see there, they determine the grade of the entire animal.

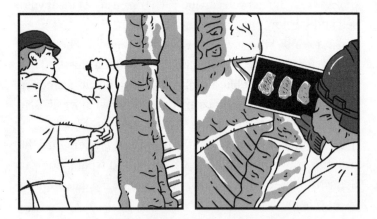

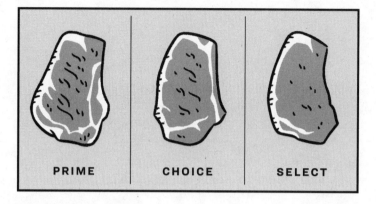

PRIME CHOICE SELECT

How is the grading done?

The inspector compares that ribeye section to photos on a "grader card." The grader card is a key that has pictures of steaks on it, visual examples of what, for example, a "Prime" steak should look like. If the amount of marbling the grader sees on the ribeye closely resembles the photo, that whole carcass will be stamped "PRIME," and the grader will move on to the next carcass. It is a quick process that takes mere seconds.

What does the grader look for?

The only thing a grader is concerned with is marbling, as the USDA considers marbling a major attribute of flavor.

How many grades are there?

There are eight grades: Prime, Choice, Select, Standard, Commercial, Utility, Cutter and Canner.

Prime: the most marbled. Approximately 3% of all graded beef in America.

Choice: moderate marbling. About 50% of graded beef sold.

Select: less marbling than Prime or Choice. Leaner, as marbling equals fat.

Standard, Commercial, Utility, Cutter and Canner: typically beef from older cattle, over forty-two months. The meat will end up in canned and processed foods, including hot dogs, bologna and beef jerky—or in cheap ground beef.

5

What Makes a Steak a Steak?

ALL STEAK is beef, but not all beef is steak, so what actually makes a steak? And why is all steak not created equal?

First, let's take a look at what we know as the proverbial side of beef. It is literally a side of beef, because the carcass is split right down the middle, along the spine. That side is made up of primals, which in turn are made up of subprimals. The common primals are the chuck, the rib, the loin, the round, the brisket, the plate and the flank. Then there is the shank, which is pretty much the lower shoulder.

Within these primals are subprimals. Inside the loin you have the shortloin, sirloin, tenderloin and top and bottom sirloin. All have different flavors and different palatabilities. Those subprimals get cut a bit further down into cuts of meat that a consumer would cook, like a roast, a pot roast, a chuck roast, a whole tenderloin—but those aren't steaks. They're whole muscle cuts.

HOW A STEAK IS BORN

SUBPRIMAL TRIMMED AND READY FOR STEAK CUTTING

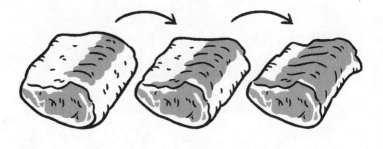

RIBEYE SUBPRIMAL READY FOR STEAKS

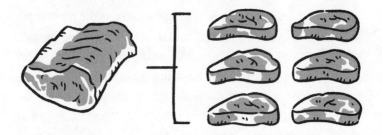

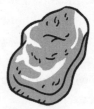

**FINAL TRIMMED
BONELESS
RIBEYE STEAK**

So what is a steak? A steak is a piece cut out of a whole muscle for an individual serving. When I take that flank and I cut it into pieces, they become steaks. When I take that rib and I cut it into ribeye steaks, they become individual servings—they become steaks.

The easiest one to think about is the tenderloin. When I take that tenderloin and cut it into filets, those filets are steaks; the rest of the tenderloin that's uncut isn't. Some people might argue that a twenty-ounce tomahawk is not a steak, because it's, well, twenty ounces, but it's still considered a steak, because it's prepared as such. It's a very, very large steak, but a steak, nonetheless. The reality is that not every steak is truly intended to be for just one person. Some of them are just too big. In fact, at my favorite steakhouse, I often ask them to split a steak and "julienne" it—slice it in diagonal pieces—and I'll share it with someone.

Now let's look at the high-end steaks and low-end steaks. Some of the high-ends are going to be from the tenderloin, which creates the filet mignon. Most people consider it the most tender—and it is. It's a very flavorful steak.

Then you have the porterhouse. It used to be called the T-bone, but no one calls it a T-bone anymore; it's now a porterhouse. On one side of the T-shaped bone is the steak that by itself would be a New York strip, and on the other side is the filet. Some purists will argue that the T-bone and the porterhouse are not the same, since the T-bone is located farther back on the animal, and the porterhouse, which is on the same part of the tenderloin, is larger. But mostly what is sold today is the porterhouse.

Then you get into what I really like, which is the ribeye. I like how marbly it is, I like that intramuscular fat, and I find it easier to prepare than most other cuts. I think I probably save the ribeye for my decadence cut. My indulgence.

Those are some of the popular high-end cuts, but cheaper cuts can also be really good. I've done a chuck steak. The chuck steak has been called the seven-bone steak because it has a lot of bones in it, but that shouldn't stop you from trying it. If you get a Choice chuck—or even if you get a Prime chuck, because they're out there—you can get a really, really good cut of meat for an incredibly low price. I'm talking $5 for a really large steak. You'd want it to be graded Choice 4 or higher, and you shouldn't expect it to taste like a filet mignon—let's not pretend it is what it isn't—but that chuck would have flavor, it would have bite, and there's nothing wrong with that. If it's prepared properly, in a way that kind of meat should be prepared—maybe you sear it, maybe you broil it or even slow cook it—the chuck steak will be very tasty. I think it's one of those really underrated pieces of meat that gets overlooked because so much chuck just gets ground into hamburger. Plus, people are so obsessed with the four big ones—filet, ribeye, top sirloin and striploin—that they skip over any other possibilities.

The chuckeye, which is the muscle deep inside the chuck, can be sliced into a steak, too. It'll be a little more expensive because of the labor involved in pulling that chuckeye out, rather than just taking the whole chuck and cutting it into steaks, but it can be done.

There are so many cuts out there that are overlooked. We can buy the high-end cuts for a good price, so we don't even bother with the others, and those cuts just end up getting ground. It's a shame. Personally, I like a lot of them and I think they're worth trying. Just put a little butter and a little salt on them and they turn out great.

But what about the beef that's not steak? There's some wonderful beef out there that's really home-and-hearth stuff: the brisket, the rump roast and the pot roast, which is usually made with chuck, are great for family meals. That being said, you've got to know what you're doing when you cook them. You've got to have some skill. Just like you'd cook a filet mignon much differently than you would cook a bone-in ribeye, the same rules apply for the cuts that aren't steaks.

But do your research. Go online. Talk to experts. Find out the best way to prepare a chuckeye or even an oxtail. Don't make the mistake of assuming all beef cooks the same way. Most people would prefer to slap a $9 ribeye on the grill (or three or four $9 ribeyes, because we're usually not eating alone), instead of taking the time to learn how to prepare the more challenging cuts. But if you have a large family and you're on a budget, you're going to want to learn, and you won't be sorry.

And even if you're not on a budget, you're still going to want to learn. When I'm in Arizona with my kids, I always do a brisket. I start with a coffee base, then I drizzle in a very mild barbeque. It's got to be slowly cooked, so the tendons can break down on their own. You can reverse sear it too, which is a great way to cook it. After you've slow cooked it, bring it down to room temperature, then half an hour before you're ready to serve it, sear the heck out of it. All the juices stay inside, you brown the exterior, and then it's perfect. There's something very homey about my family brisket. Everyone's at the table, the aroma is wafting in the air, and my kids can absolutely polish off a five- or six-pound brisket in one sitting. If not, they end up picking at it all the next day, like a Thanksgiving turkey. They love it.

Whether it's steak, roast or brisket, it's important to know and appreciate the beef you're eating. The more you get to know it, the more it will reward you.

What Is Aged Beef?

YOU MAY have seen "aged beef" on menus but didn't know exactly what that meant. Well, just like aged cheese is considered to be tastier, aged beef is considered to be tastier, too. The point of aging meat is to bring out a beefier, more intense flavor.

There is dry aging and wet aging, and the two are entirely different processes.

Dry aging is an "age-old" method that is relatively uncommon these days. In this process, the meat is hung in a refrigerated room. It's critical that this space, this *dry-aging room*, is well ventilated, because that will control the bacteria. The temperature also must be well monitored, as it cannot go above 36°F or the meat will spoil, and if it dips below freezing the aging process will be halted. Further, the dry-aging room has to be kept humid so that the meat is kept moist. Otherwise, there will be too much water loss.

As the beef hangs in this chamber, a fungus will grow on the outside of it, which is a great tenderizer and a great flavor sealant. That fungus is there because what is happening is a controlled decomposition of the beef. It may not sound appetizing, but that's exactly what's happening.

Dry aging is an expensive endeavor. There is more yield loss on dry-aged beef, and monitoring the process takes knowledge, time and a keen eye, not to mention the expense of having and maintaining a dry-aging room. All of that costs money, which is why there isn't a lot of dry-aged beef available.

The whole process usually takes anywhere from fourteen to thirty days, and it will usually be done at high-end butcher shops or high-end restaurants. Some places will age it even longer than thirty days. The true believers will age it for months, but the longer the meat ages, the higher the risk that the meat will spoil. Also, there aren't a lot of people who enjoy the taste of meat that's been aged for so long. Dry aging changes the flavor of beef because, just like with cheese, the chemical composition of the beef is changing and enzymes are breaking down the proteins. As a result of that process, the texture of the beef will be very velvety and the meat will be very tender, too tender for a lot of palates.

In my opinion, nobody ages beef better than my friend and partner Ray Rastelli, who has a giant dry-aging chamber at his plant. He thinks of aged beef as having a nuttier flavor. It's more intense and more aromatic, and the meat is denser. "It definitely is a bit more of an acquired taste," says Rastelli. "Not everyone likes it. For many people, it's just too much for them."

Wet aging is how most of the beef in the United States is aged. The process is a pretty simple one. The beef is shipped in Cryovac packages and will be refrigerated in these packages for a couple of weeks, which is how the beef ages. In a Cryovac, the meat is packed tight in its own juices, in an oxygen-free container. This allows the enzymes to break down the connective tissue, which makes the meat more tender. There is no evaporation as there is in dry aging, so there is not the accompanying yield loss. The vast majority of meat in this country is wet aged.

When I see "aged beef" on a menu, I'm skeptical. That doesn't tell me if it was wet aged or dry aged, or if it's just old meat, which it absolutely is sometimes. It's important to remember that wet aged is very common and dry aged is uncommon. If the beef is dry aged, the butcher or the restaurant is going to want to show that off. They're going to want to promote this process that they've invested so much in. They will be highly knowledgeable about the process and offer to tell you about it, or provide a detailed description on their menu.

So if you're looking at the menu and all you see is "aged beef," with no other information or added details, be leery. It could just be old meat.

7

What Should the Cow You're Eating Be Eating?

F OR COWS, it's all about the grass. As far as they're concerned, it's really the only thing that should be on the menu. But this is not lawn grass I'm talking about. These are grasses that are grown in pastures, and I'd say the top grasses for cattle are bluegrass, timothy, ryegrass, Bermuda, foxtail and sorghum-sudangrass. There are a lot of non-grass plants in pastures, too, that are highly nutritious. There's alfalfa, vetch, red and white clover and other sources of naturally occurring vegetation that are great for cattle.

For most of their lives, this is all cattle eat. Some might dine in better meadows than others, where the grass is greener and tastier than the dried-up fields over in the next state, but they all eat grass. Grass for breakfast, grass for lunch, grass for dinner and grass for snacks when they're bored and there's nothing on Netflix. When they go to sleep, they dream about the grass they'll eat when they wake up. When they wake up, they start eating it.

Grass is to cows what sunshine is to flowers: they just need it. They are a grazing creature by nature. They don't need to be trained to do it; it's instinctive. This is as true of the cow in Colombia as it is of the cow in Iceland, Mongolia, Russia, Austria, America or anywhere else cows are heard mooing. The bovine belly was specially designed to digest grass and little else, so guess what? That's what they eat.

Except when they don't. In America, the majority of cattle are put on high rations of corn, combined with silage, for the last few months before heading to slaughter. This is what they finish on. But that wasn't always the case.

Corn wasn't commonly used in American cattle feed until after World War II, when farmers had an abundance of the grain and no one to sell it to. They had harvested vast amounts of it to feed soldiers cheap chow, but with those soldiers back home and hungry for beef instead of an Army-issued dollop of Spam, the farmers eventually figured out that if they fed the excess corn crop to the cattle, they could fatten the cows fast and get more beef onto American plates. Win-win.

But a cow would no sooner eat a kernel of corn than it would eat a peacock feather, so the grain was pulverized to make it appetizing. Once the farmer saw his cattle gobbling up the powdery meal, he realized he didn't have to produce quality corn. He could get away with any old thing. So he began to grow low-grade corn, and still does today. Some of it is *very* low grade. The corn that cattle consume bears little resemblance to the corn we eat. There's no way we would be able to stomach the grain that the cattle get. So let's be clear: there is cow corn and there is people corn.

Milo, which is a type of sorghum, is also dumped into the feed. So are barley and oats. Bakery waste is in the mix, too, which is pretty much anything that's swept up off the floor— apple pomace, ingredients left over from cereal, granola bars, breads. Oilseeds like soy and canola are also dumped in because they really help to aid digestion of these otherwise utterly undigestible foods. All of this feedstuff is considered the silage, or ration as some people call it, and it is ground up together with the corn and dumped into the trough.

The cattle fatten really quickly eating all that sugar and starch, just like you would. And since they're shoulder to shoulder, there's nowhere to roam and burn off the calories, so they just gain and gain. They're vertical couch potatoes. The only thing missing is a TV remote. This is how the majority of American beef cattle are fed the last few months before slaughter.

The remaining minority are finished on grass. This means these cows aren't herded to the feedlot like their corn-fed cousins. Instead, they stay on the pastures and continue to munch on the green stuff. It takes longer for them to reach their optimal weight, not only because they aren't eating calorie-heavy feed, but also because they're still walking off their meals.

So what should cattle be finished on: corn or grass? That depends. Are you talking about how it's going to affect flavor, or are you talking about what's best for your health?

Let's start with your health, because that's a quick and easy answer, and the answer is grass. That grass-fed cow will be a healthier animal. It won't become morbidly obese, because it wasn't crammed onto a feedlot and forced to eat food for which its stomach wasn't designed. And it also won't be exposed to the other questionable items that are dumped into the troughs of corn-fed cattle—mainly hormones and antibiotics.

All that good grass eating, right up to the finish line, produces beef that is five times higher in omega-3, and omega-3 is so badass it should be wearing a cape. It's a fatty acid known to fight killers like heart disease, cancer and diabetes. But you need to know that the beef from the grass-finished cow will have little marbling, that prized intramuscular fat so ubiquitous on the corn-fed cow. That marbling got there because that cow pigged out on the sugary, starchy corn for a couple of months straight, and barely lifted a muscle doing it. In this country, fat equals flavor. The American palate has been trained to salivate over it.

So if it's purely the flavor experience you're after— the fattypalooza, loosen-your-belt, molten-chocolate-cake indulgence—you're probably going to want the cow that's been corn-fed. This is Saturday-night-at-the-steakhouse gluttony, when you have your favorite bourbon in front of you and your favorite ribeye on your plate, and you don't care about your ticker lasting till its sell-by date. You just want the molten chocolate cake. This is when you push away the fruit salad, pat your belly and dig in.

I'm here to tell you, though, that grass-fed can be every bit as indulgent as corn-fed. With grass-finished cattle, you have to understand that you're tasting more of the meat than the fat. The flavor tends to be more nuanced and will reflect much more specifically where the cattle was raised—the grasses of Iowa taste different than the grasses of Texas, and your tongue can tell. Some say grass-finished beef has a gamey taste, but I don't agree. In Europe, the majority of cattle are grass-finished cattle, and one of the best beef experiences I've ever had in my life was in Rome. The waiter knew as much about the steak as he did about the wine. He knew the farmer, the diet, the age. It was a delicious Piedmontese, and entirely grass-fed.

I tend to look at it this way: Back when I was growing up, ice-cold Budweiser was the perfect indulgence after a long day of work. I can still hear the snap of the pop-top on the can. I can still taste that first guzzle. It was the signal that it was the end of the day and now it was time to relax. At some point, Corona became everyone's basic go-to brew, but what also happened was IPAs. They matured our palates. They awoke our senses to a whole range of nuance and subtlety. In some ways, I view grass-fed the same way. We didn't know until recently that there was a world of taste beyond the conventional corn-fed beef we grew up on.

When I'm talking about flavor, I can't just say, "This cow was corn-fed, so it must be a real crowd-pleaser, and this cow was grass-fed, so the flavor is muted." There are many factors affecting taste. What the cow ate is just one of them.

But it is a big one.

8

What's Good about Your Beef?

I N 1980, the USDA, together with the Department of Health and Human Services, published its first "Dietary Guidelines for Americans," in which it had more to say about what not to do than what to do: don't get fat, don't eat foods high in fat and cholesterol, don't eat too much sugar, don't consume too much sodium, don't drink too much alcohol, eat foods with adequate starch and fiber and eat a variety of foods.

They also threw in a handy chart to show the ballpark number of calories that could be burned in an hour of various activities (sleeping: 80; chopping wood: 400). This was sourced by a seemingly random guy named Robert Johnson, a doctor at University of Illinois. I imagine Bob and his cohorts coming up with these over cigarettes and coffee in the breakroom. They estimated square dancing to burn 350 calories an hour. They threw in domestic work, whatever they presumed that entailed, as burning only 180 per hour. (Clearly, Bob had never lugged a 1980s-era Electrolux vacuum cleaner up and down a flight of stairs.) But overall, that was the extent of the guidelines. It was eighteen pages with a lot of white space and a lot of charts and graphs.

Twenty-five years later, the booklet had expanded to include seventy-one pages and forty-one recommendations. The current edition comes in at 149 pages, and I suspect there will be far more in the release that follows that one.

One of the items on its current list is how much beef should be eaten, and that guideline has currently come to rest at a three-ounce portion, two or three times a week. (When you think of a three-ounce steak, think about the size of a deck of playing cards.) This isn't much. Imagine being told you didn't need more than three ounces of veggies a few times a week. But it just goes to show you that beef is a nutritional powerhouse.

Honestly, we were built to eat beef. We were given two arms and two legs—ideal for hunting and gathering—and a gut filled with three pounds of bacteria lying in wait to process all manner of foodstuff, not the least of which is meat. We eat fruit. We eat legumes. We eat vegetables. We can digest everything from tree bark to Oreo cookies. Yet, it's beef we adore, and if we don't slather it in butter, render it in a pound of its own fat, burn it like a Coppertoned butt and suck it down at every meal, beef is a healthy food.

First, there's the protein factor, and it's important to note that not all proteins are created equal. Depending on the cut, a three-ounce portion of beef should provide half of the daily requirement of protein. Plant-based proteins don't come with all of the amino acids your body needs, but red meat does. This is important, because amino acids—the ones your body makes on its own and the ones it can only get from an outside source, like beef—are critical for your body. They're the great synthesizers. They help your cells grow, and they help produce neurotransmitters, like serotonin and melatonin. They help protect your heart by making nitric oxide, which helps lower blood pressure. Protein is the body's support system. It does everything from keeping your cells in good shape, to keeping your bones strong, to giving a boost to your immune system.

Then there's iron. That three-ounce steak will provide 20 percent of the daily iron requirements for men and 10 percent for women. Iron aids brain function and muscle function. It produces red blood cells, transports oxygen all over the body and equalizes body temperature. It's a mineral critical to maintaining good health, and—bonus for beef eaters—the iron in red meat is easier for the body to synthesize than the iron provided by plants.

Red meat has nearly the entire B-complex body of vitamins. (There are scores of B vitamins, and eight of them are collectively known as B-complex: thiamine (B_1), riboflavin (B_2), niacin (B_3), pantothenic acid (B_5), pyridoxine (B_6), biotin (B_7), folate (B_9) and cobalamin (B_{12}).) They all have unique functions to human health, but a large part of the job is to aid healthy digestion, in part by effectively eliminating toxins. Plus, they're packed with antioxidants.

Zinc is another important mineral we get from red meat. It's a super immune booster, it's great for brain health and it helps keep inflammatory diseases at bay. The average

American needs somewhere around ten milligrams of zinc each day. That three-ounce steak will provide approximately half of that.

Beef also has generous amounts of phosphorus, which helps us absorb B vitamins; potassium, the great regulator of blood pressure; and magnesium, the calming mineral that helps boost energy levels, at the same time allowing the body to better relax.

And it has omega-3, which, as I've already said, is badass. That three-ounce steak will have eighty milligrams of omega-3 if it's grass-finished. This is around 10 percent of the daily requirement, but still a good start. Grass-fed also has an overall lower fat-to-protein ratio than its grain-fed cousin, which means fewer calories.

Grass-fed beef contains significantly higher levels of vitamins A, K, D, E and CLA, a type of omega-6 that helps regulate the metabolic rate and lower cholesterol.

But not all beef is created equal. The nutritional value depends on a variety of factors, including the size of the portion, how it's prepared and even the cut of the beef. Further, Americans consume almost half of their red meat as ground beef, and ground beef can be high in saturated and trans fat.

By law, though, ground beef cannot contain more than 30 percent fat. Most ground beef has the lean-to-fat ratio printed right on the packaging, If the package indicates 70/30, that means the ground beef has the maximum fat content allowed by law. To truly qualify as "lean" in the eyes of the USDA, the ground beef cannot contain more than 22.5 percent fat. "Extra lean" can have no more than 15 percent fat.

(Hot dogs, on the other hand, are not bound by the same legal requirement as ground beef, so they can have more fat—the ratio will probably be around 60/40.)

However, it's important to be mindful that the cuts that went into the ground beef will not necessarily translate into leaner beef. For example, if a package of ground beef states that the meat is "ground sirloin," and you know that sirloin is traditionally a lean cut, that ground beef will not necessarily be leaner than ground beef made from a mix of cuts. It may well be, but it's not a given. The ratio on the package will be the best guide.

If you're conscientious about what and how you're eating—portion size, fat content, preparation—beef cannot be beat for nutritional value. But even the most health-conscious beef eater should be aware that there are aspects of beef production that affect quality long before that beef gets to the table. We'll get to those next.

9

What's Bad about Your Beef?

Y OU NEED to know how lean your beef is. You need to
know what the cattle was fed. But you also need to know
what else was in the feed and what else the cattle were
given, because there is a lot that goes on at the feedlot
that can affect your choices.

Let's take a look.

The vast majority of feedlots in America are pretty small
operations. They are licensed to provide feed for up to a thousand head of cattle. Believe it or not, a thousand head of cattle
is a small operation. Some of them will have half that, maybe
450 head of cattle, or even fewer.

Then there are the big feedlots, the ones with thousands
and thousands of cattle, and while these large operations make
up less than 5 percent of the feedlots in this country, they are
responsible for a whopping 85 percent of feed cattle. Eighty-
five percent! The largest in the world is Five Rivers Cattle

Feeding, which has close to a million head of cattle on eleven feedlots spread out across the Midwest. Many, many feedlots have 160,000 cows—or more. That's triple the seating capacity of Yankee Stadium, without the space. That's larger than the population of Charleston, South Carolina, without the space. And that's Big Beef. These big packers know they need to do whatever they can do to keep profits high and expenses low, and overcrowded feedlots are their current solution.

Cattle are packed into a tight space so they'll gain faster. A roaming cow is a pound-dropping cow, and that costs the feeder money. So the cattle aren't encouraged to roam. Instead, they are bellied up to the trough like drunks to a bar, and as long as that feed is coming down the line, they'll stand there and eat it. They've gotten used to being shoulder to shoulder, and they have a Pavlovian response whenever they hear that feed wagon trundling up. They're thinking, "Yum, someone's gonna drop some sugary neat stuff in there, and it's gonna be good." Meanwhile, the whole time they're eating, they're standing in their own shit. Because, as I said, there's no place to roam, and they don't get bathroom breaks.

With feedlots that have more than 160,000 head of cattle—and some that have nearly a million—that's a lot of urine and a lot of fecal matter. The crap gets shoveled away, but not always fast enough. There's a big opportunity for disease spread.

Humans couldn't live like that. If forty people were crammed into a home and given one toilet and one sink and were fed from one area all at the same time, everyone would get sick. No question. But that's essentially how a feedlot operates. So of course the cattle are given preventive antibiotics. If they weren't, death loss would be high. And it's in the economic interest not to have that.

Approximately 80 percent of all antibiotics sold in the United States are used on livestock. This number is disputed by the beef industry, but it holds up under scrutiny. The percentage was arrived at by combining FDA data on sales of antibiotics for use on "food-producing animals" and projected sales of antibiotics to humans. Both the Johns Hopkins Bloomberg School of Public Health and the Pew Research Center crunched the same numbers and validated the report.

Now listen, these major cattle-feeding operations do their best to keep the pens clean. When cattle are moved, let's say on to slaughter, there is usually a solid washdown of the concrete they've been standing on, which has a non-slip groove. This is typically done before a new batch of cattle are moved to that pen. But no one is inspecting or regulating on a daily basis to make sure this is done.

Joel Salatin, a farmer and lecturer who is at the vanguard of grass-fed farming, says you need to respect the cowness of the cow and the chickenness of the chicken. What do these animals look like in their normal conditions and surroundings? What should a cow be doing all day, and what should a chicken be doing all day? Certainly not eating from a cup or a plastic bucket and inhaling particulate fecal matter.

There are a ton of diseases that come out of factory farms. The animals contract everything from mastitis to anthrax. So when a conventional farmer spots a sick cow or two, he will usually treat the whole herd. It wouldn't make sense for him to have a veterinarian check each and every animal. That would be time consuming and expensive. So he drops amoxicillin or tetracycline or whatever is called for on all of them. That's a lot of antibiotics. Quite a lot. More than thirty-four million pounds of antibiotics were sold for veterinary use in 2015 (the most recent year of FDA data). Compare that with more than seven million pounds for the American population.

But animals aren't just fed antibiotics for disease prevention. For decades, farmers have also been using them to promote growth.

During the golden age of antibiotics in the 1950s and 1960s, farmers were delighted to discover that when they gave antibiotics to a member of their herd, that cow fattened quicker than the others.

For years previous to this, farmers had been struggling with how to keep up with the increasing demand for meat. They had tried fattening their livestock with cod liver oil and fish meal (when feeding cattle animal byproducts was still permitted). That worked, because both of these substances contain animal proteins, which are essential to producing measurable gain. But that was about the only thing that worked. They tried all manner of vegetable proteins, but nothing was as good as cod liver oil and fish meal. The only problem was that those two items had to be imported from Japan, which was costly. When World War II came, it became impossible.

In the late 1940s, it so happened that scientists at the pharmaceutical company Merck were looking for a treatment for a particular type of anemia. It had been known for some time that eating liver could cure the disease, but it was Merck researchers who were able to isolate the heroic substance animal liver produced, and that substance was vitamin B_{12}. Soon after that discovery, they developed the ability to synthesize the vitamin.

The fortuitous and extremely accidental link for American farmers came a couple of years later, when a different group of scientists fed B_{12} to a group of chickens to see if the vitamin would enhance their health. Not only did it enhance the health of the chickens, but there were unexpected, nearly comical results the farmers could not have foreseen, but were delighted by. Their chickens were turning into some kind of growth action heroes. They gained and gained. A closer look revealed why: it wasn't the B_{12} giving them the miracle, it was the synthesizing antibiotic, Aureomycin, which happened to be lacing the vitamin.

Farmers tried it on other livestock. They gave antibiotics to some cows, and those cows fattened fast. It was a bonanza moment for them, a time to throw out the pitchfork and dance around the barn, because it was as good as finding a mint to make their own money. They were quite caught up in their mirth and their money, and no one apparently alerted them to the warning in the *New England Journal of Medicine*, which in the sixties raised the alarm about overuse of antibiotics. "Bacterial resistance," the report stated, would put civilization "back in the pre-antibiotic Middle Ages."

As word spread up the troughline about this quick-gain tip, more and more farmers started to add antibiotics to the feedlot regimen, regardless of whether or not the herd was sick. Quicker than a cow can moo, it became a practice so standard farmers could hardly a remember a day when it hadn't been done. The farmers would put a low-dose antibiotic into the water, and all the way down the line, the cattle would dip their fat tongues in and lap it up.

The type of antibiotic the farmers used is called an ionophore, and ionophores don't kill bacteria. What they do is they stifle bacteria. Think of an ionophore as "It" in freeze tag: When an ionophore tags certain bacteria, those bacteria can no longer reproduce. And they can't function the way they had done before they were targeted.

This type of antibiotic is very specific about the bacteria it goes after and has a unique effect on corn-fed cattle. Here's why: A bovine stomach is like a complicated factory floor, made up of four compartments. One of them is called the rumen, which is where volatile fatty acids are produced. Those fatty acids provide energy for the cow. But the problem comes when you introduce things like grains, because the cow's stomach wasn't designed for grains. The stomach was designed for grass. It's like putting diesel in a gas-fueled car.

Eating grain upsets the balance between two key fatty acids, acetate and propionate. It produces much more acetate than the bovine body needs and throws the pH levels way off. These two, acetate and propionate, should work in tandem to produce energy for the cow (along with a third, called butyrate, which is unaffected by a grain-based diet), but since they don't, the cow's body spends energy—meaning it burns calories—trying to compensate for the imbalance. The ionophores come to the rescue, because they don't just affect bacteria, they also "freeze tag" the extra acetate fatty acids. Balance restored, the cow can continue to eat and gain, unhindered by the fuss going on in its belly.

This is all irrelevant to the grass-finished cow, which, in normal circumstances, maintains a Buddha-like balance in its belly. Why? Because it's eating what comes naturally to it. Those farmers back in the fifties and sixties weren't really seeing weight gain. What they were seeing was how little their cattle were gaining when fed corn, as compared with what the cattle gained on grass. Corn was such an inefficient fuel for the cattle that the animals had to spend a lot more energy trying to convert it. The ionophore antibiotics only came in as an equalizer. Adding antibiotics to cattle feed quickly became the thing to do. Ionophores were used generously and daily, and no farmer could afford not to dole it out to his herds. That would be like trying to compete clean against Lance Armstrong in the Tour de France. In this sense, ionophores are cow doping.

The practice went unchecked for about twenty years. Everyone ignored the *New England Journal of Medicine*'s warning, and it wasn't until the late 1970s that the FDA tried to ban the use of antibiotics for growth in livestock. It cited a threat to public health, stating that the more antibiotics are used, the less effective they are in humans.

Think about it. If large herds are consuming large quantities of antibiotics, they are also crapping it out. That crap either ends up as manure for your vegetables or winds up in the waterways of the fish you eat. So you're not just getting those antibiotics in your meat, they are getting spread over everything. Nevertheless, Congress blocked the FDA back in 1979 from doing anything about it. But the FDA continued to soldier on, and after forty-four years, it finally won the battle. If all goes as scheduled, the FDA says that ionophores will no longer be allowed in cattle feed by mid-2023.

Honestly, we might just owe our salvation to a group of nuns, rather than the FDA. The Congregation of Benedictine Sisters in Boerne, Texas, sounded the horn so loud about live-stock antibiotics, it shook corporate heads. The sisters have a watchdog system, in which they go around buying shares in companies they feel need policing. As shareholders of McDonald's (and Denny's and Sanderson Farms), the sisters filed resolutions calling on the corporations to ensure all their beef was free of antibiotics.

Years before the sisters took action, McDonald's had decided to go antibiotic-free with its chicken, although not its beef. But within a year after the nuns put pressure on them as shareholders, McDonald's agreed to reduce antibiotics in their beef. Those are some pretty awesome nuns.

But what does "reduce antibiotics" even mean? You could remove one cow from the herd and not feed it antibiotics and that's a reduction. You could lessen the dosage by a half per-cent, and that would be a reduction. And if McDonald's does reduce antibiotics by any measurable standard, how will it be proven? What governing body or organization will provide the checks and balances? And what reduction is enough? Ten percent? Twenty percent? Sixty percent? And says who? To date, none of this has been addressed.

It's not just about the antibiotics, either. It's also about the hormones. Around the same time farmers discovered the trick ionophores could pull, they found out what hormones could do for the herd. Hormone injections gave steers back the testosterone they would have gotten naturally had they stayed bulls, and heifers were often given an extra dose of estrogen to speed them along. Soon, the FDA approved a list of several hormones that could be used in American cattle, and it's been that way ever since. A hormone-injected calf can get up to a 20 percent gain over one that's not been injected, which means more profit for the beef industrial complex. All it takes is a small pellet inserted under the skin on the back flap of one ear, and voila, a slow, steady drip to make the calf grow faster and bigger.

But hormones aren't used just to get bigger cows. Farmers mix and match like scientists in a very large lab to get the results they want. Cattle can be fattened with one hormone, or made leaner with another, and behavior-modified with yet another.

The question is whether hormones given to cattle are safe— for the cattle or for the humans. The European Union banned American hormone-treated beef more than thirty years ago, concluding a link to cancer, although the World Trade Organization shot back that the EU had insufficient data for such a claim. It has remained a big international food fight, but so far the EU is still winning. And good for them for sticking to their guns.

The controversy is the same on American turf: Is hormone-treated beef bad for you? The FDA says no. Opponents say it can cause a host of problems, ranging from early onset puberty to cancer.

The current policy is that cattle must be off both antibiotics and hormones for the last ninety days before slaughter, but can we really say that's sufficient? It should be clear by now that you can't separate animal welfare from human welfare. The use of antibiotics and hormones is one of the biggest controversies currently facing the conventional beef industry.

Hey, let's not fool anyone. I eat conventional beef sometimes. Yes, I co-founded what is now the largest organic beef company in the United States, but I'll still occasionally eat conventional beef. It's probably what I'm always eating when I order steak off a menu, and I eat out a lot. And I eat a lot of beef. But at least I know what I'm eating. I believe you have the right to know, too. You have a right to know what you're eating, to know where it came from and to make your own decisions based on that.

10

The Life and Times of a Beef Cow

A N OLD cow tastes about as good as an old shoe, and this is why the lives of quality beef cattle are kept very brief, lasting, on average, eighteen to twenty-two months. Certainly no longer than thirty months. During that lifespan, they will spend time on pastures and in feedlots—but mostly in feedlots—and be bought and sold at least three times before they end up at the packing plant.

Here's a look at the stages of a beef cow's life.

Stage one: The cow-calfer

American cattle that are bound to wind up as steak start out life in the care of what's called a cow-calfer. This is a farmer, still typically a guy, who owns a herd of mother cows that, with any luck, will each give birth once a year (cows have the same gestation period as humans). The cow-calfer has a few bulls on hand to do the job of getting them pregnant, some of whom he's kept and raised. But he will also purchase bulls, and for that he will rely on his practiced eye and the long tradition of the "Rancher's Religion": going to auction and sizing up which is the prized bull to sire the best calves. These guys can eyeball a bull and know just from looking at it whether it's going to produce offspring that are Prime, Choice or Select. There's no way to quantify it; they're just good at it. But what it comes down to, the key attributes they look for, are a flat back, a big chest and a big butt. If a bull has those three features, there's a good chance he's considered a prized bull.

Usually, this top bull has been fattened up far beyond what's practical, just for the pomp and splendor of showcasing him at auction. He'll be too obese to mount a cow without crippling himself, so the cow-calfer will have to put his boy on a diet before he's ready for the work. Once the bull has slimmed down a bit, he's ready to go, and he and his other bull buddies on the ranch will each be expected to impregnate twenty or thirty cows a year.

When the cow-calfer's not relying on his practiced eye, he's relying on a pricey vial. Bovine artificial insemination has been around for nearly seventy years, but it's used in beef cattle only about 10 percent of the time. A very expensive vial of bull semen, purchased from a very wealthy bovine genetics specialist, or seedstock producer, will cost upwards of $80,000. It's nothing more than a frozen straw of bull seed, yet it costs a bundle—but one vial of frozen semen can impregnate hundreds of cows, which can be well worth the steep upfront cost.

How is it used? The cow-calfer just walks over to the cow, lifts her tail, squirts the bull's best in her and that's it, she's pregnant. She doesn't even get a goodnight kiss.

Once the calves are born, they stick close to their moms for a long while. They feed from her udders until they eventually learn to forage and graze on their own, which happens at around six months of age. At birth, they weigh anywhere from sixty to one hundred pounds, but they'll be tipping the scale toward 450 pounds by the time they're weaned.

All of the initial health checks are done at the cow-calfer's, and the vet will give any of the vaccinations the state requires. Most of the male calves will be castrated, as steers make superior meat to bulls, and, of course, they're far more compliant.

Stage two: The backgrounder

When the calves are fully weaned from their moms, they're often sold to a "backgrounder." This is usually a fat-cat rancher with a whole lot of land. Those cows you see when you're out on your country drive? The ones lazily grazing in bucolic pastures? They are on this guy's property.

Out in the meadows, the cattle do nothing but roam and graze and drink fresh water and flutter their long eyelashes under warm summer suns. The roaming is important because it builds bone and muscle, and the relaxing is good because a stressed animal is an unhealthy animal. When winter comes, being out in the pasture is no problem, because cows are warm-blooded and like the cold. They stay out there and eat the hay the backgrounder has prepared for them. But too cold is too cold, so when the mercury really dips, the backgrounder shelters them.

They spend maybe nine months with the backgrounder, and by the time they are sold off again, they weigh in at half a ton. Bovines are bought and sold by weight, so if the backgrounder bought a calf for, say, $2 a pound and sold that same animal for $2 a pound but at twice the weight, he doubled his money in less than a year and got his grass mowed for free. And he's not just buying one calf, he's buying a good many. They will background both steers and heifers (female cows who've never given birth), and by the time the herd has grown from calves to feeder cattle, the fat-cat rancher has turned a very tidy profit.

Now listen, all of this is true, but it's all getting less true. In a lot of cases, those calves go right into a feedlot. They skip their time with the backgrounder and, therefore, their time in the pasture. In the world of cattle, the backgrounder is becoming less and less prominent, and unless you're doing grass-fed or organic, where you're required by the USDA to have the animal on pasture a specified amount of time, don't count on the cattle getting any time with a backgrounder.

Stage three (or, as I just said, sometimes stage two): The feedlot

Once the cattle get to the feedlot, they eat from troughs, not pastures, and have a far more confined space. The reason for this is for the cattle to add about three hundred more pounds in three months—topping off at 1,300 pounds before they're ready for slaughter—and they can't pack on the pounds if they're walking miles a day like they did in the backgrounder's pastures.

And that's about it. There are variances, of course. None of this is set in stone, and sadly, some might say, more and more calves are heading straight to the feedlot.

11

All You Never Wanted to Know about Processing

N O ONE who eats meat really likes to think about the processing. We'd rather not be reminded that what we're buying and what we're eating once had a face, four legs and a tail that gently wagged. Unless you live in an area where hunters abound, you probably grew up getting your meat from a butcher or a grocery store chain. You never thought about the animal and you liked it that way.

For its part, the industry has done a lot to remove you from that animal in the language they use. We don't eat cow, we eat beef. We don't eat pig, we eat bacon or pork. You'll never see a label that reads "grass-fed cow," it's always "grass-fed beef." How can beef eat grass? It's impossible! Beef can't eat anything. Beef isn't even alive. The day beef grows lips and eats grass is the day my bathrobe gets up and runs a marathon.

Yet, you see the "grass-fed beef" label so often, you don't even question the fact that it makes no sense. That wording is very consciously designed to create a distance between what you put in your mouth and what once *had* a mouth.

I would guess the reason the lamb industry has struggled in the United States is because there's no good name for the meat. No one wants to eat a cute little lamb. We call turkey "turkey," and we call chicken "chicken," but then we've also been led to believe that turkeys and chickens are really stupid, even though the reality is they have complex emotional natures, individual personalities and a capacity for empathy and self-control—indicators of solid cognitive abilities. But the chicken industry is happy to have us go on thinking that these birds are dumb, because if we do, then our own empathy response won't kick in.

But what all of these animals have in common is that they've been selectively bred to feed people. The chicken that exists today was specifically bred to be a broiler. You could not release that chicken to live in the wild for more than thirty minutes. It was bred to eat and to gain and to have big breasts. Other countries do it, too. There are turkeys in Algeria that weigh forty-five pounds or more. When you drive past the turkey farms, you can see small mountains of feathers. It looks like a feather pillow factory exploded. The birds are specifically engineered for the restaurant industry and are so enormous they have to be cooked in a baker's oven. They won't fit in a conventional oven. But the turkey is delicious, the best you'll ever eat.

If these birds had their way, surely they'd envy the skinny turkeys and their free will. But that's not the life they were bred for, and that's not the life most American cattle were bred for, either. They were bred to feed a nation. It bears repeating that nearly a hundred thousand head of cattle are slaughtered every day in America. That's almost three million cows a month. That's a lot of steak. That's a lot of hamburger.

I think it's important for you to know how those cows are processed. Knowing what goes on behind the scenes, knowing how your beef becomes beef, will unyoke you from the masses of buyers who just sling their package of ground beef into the grocery cart before they head to the condiments aisle without ever giving a thought to the fact that the ground beef used to be part of a living, breathing animal.

Here's how it happens:

Cattle get delivered to their final fate at night, in a truck with about thirty or thirty-five other animals. They are going to a holding facility, and by the time they get delivered there, the animals have been on the truck anywhere up to ten hours. The bigger packing houses that are killing up to a thousand head per hour are going to have huge holding facilities where they can store enough animals to slaughter in one shift.

After the cow is off-loaded, it is going to sit in another holding facility with other animals from all over the country. They are all held overnight, and in the morning, usually around six or seven a.m., they're lined up to go down a chute, which is sometimes jokingly called the "Stairway to Heaven."

After the cow goes down the chute, it'll be led into what's called a knocking box. It walks into this knocking box (or, in some cases, is moved along an escalator, like a moving sidewalk at the airport) and puts its head through a small hole, and the box kind of closes in on the animal. There's a butt push that pushes the animal forward so it can't move. Think of it as a kind of cow guillotine. The point of the knocking box is to knock the cow out. It's where it gets stunned with a high-powered stun gun. The standard way to stun an animal is a reciprocating bolt into the head, which is basically an electric or .22 caliber bolt that shoots about two inches into the skull of the cow. The target is about three inches above its eyes, right where there's a tuft of hair. That is the bull's-eye for the "knocker," and the stun gun is fired right into that spot.

At this point, the animal is not killed, it's stunned. It's rolled out to the left onto what's called the kill floor. Its hind legs are shackled and then lifted up in the air, at which time a butcher holding a very sharp knife, a guy we call the knocker, slices the carotid artery, opens the throat up and bleeds the animal out. And that's when it dies. It's considered painless. I don't know. I'm not a cow. But typically, if you do it right and you're good at it, there's very little reaction, very little stress. The whole process from entering the knocking box to bleeding out is extremely swift. From the time of the butt push to death is seconds. If it takes more than ten seconds, something's wrong.

To bleed it out takes around twenty to thirty seconds. Remember, this is a factory, so they're not doing this one at a time. There are a lot of cattle getting bled out at the same time. The blood drains down into a collection tank and is then put into a blood truck and shipped off. The blood gets used in a multitude of ways, but some of it ends up as blood meal fertilizer. There is zero waste at a packing facility because there is no room for waste—in terms of both profit margin and physical space.

If we get in our own "wayback machine" and go back to the mid-1850s, when our waterways were even bigger dumping grounds than they are today, a lot of the carcasses ended up there. It was a hazard then, and would be an impossible situation today, with half a million head of cattle a week getting killed. That's a lot of carcasses. So every last part of the animal is reborn into something else. It goes into pet food and back into animal feed. The bones are ground up into bonemeal and burned for fuel. The blood is used not only in fertilizer, but also in cosmetics and pharmaceuticals. If they could figure out what to do with the moo, they'd profit from that, too. Sometimes I wonder what it's like for vegans to navigate a world in which dead animal dust is sprinkled on everything you touch, wear, eat, drive and breathe.

So once the blood has drained, the carcass is turned upside down. It's on a moving line, an assembly line, with guys stationed overhead. These guys are called hock cutters. As the animal moves down the line, one cutter takes the back legs off at the knee joint, and one takes the front legs off. It is then moved over and split up the stomach and gutted. All of the innards are dumped into what's called a gut buggy. Everything is opened on it—lungs, liver, spleen, gall bladder, stomach—and all of this together we call the paunch.

All of that paunch, all of the guts, gets inspected by a USDA inspector who is on site. They look for adhesions in the lungs. They look for problems with the liver. They look for anything that would cause anyone to think that the animal could have been sick. They look for any appearance that it was unhealthy in any way and, therefore, not fit for human consumption. They look at every possible aspect to decide if that animal is going to continue to be processed.

If they see any adhesions in the lungs, any concerns in any of the organs, any signs of kidney disease, for example, that animal will be tagged right there. It will be pulled off the line and put into a separate section, where it is hung and labeled "Suspect." It will not go into the food supply. It will more than likely be condemned. Now, that doesn't happen a lot. The overwhelming majority of carcasses are going to head down the line. But only healthy carcasses are ever processed. The USDA starts the inspection process here with incredible detail.

After the guts have been inspected, the animal goes to what's called a hide puller, where the hide is removed. The hide is basically peeled from the tail to the head, and it's done in such a way that it can be preserved and used as a leather product. And now you have your carcass.

The hide-puller operator, who will have a USDA inspector right next to him, will trim and clean that carcass really well. He's going to clean it using high-powered lights to spot literally anything. Any foreign material that might be on the carcass—a piece of leftover hide, dirt from the hide, anything at all—will show up under lights and be completely cleaned off.

Afterward, the carcass will go to the bandsaw, where it is then split right down the spinal cord and cut into a literal side of beef. That side of beef goes into what is called a Chad cabinet (named after the manufacturer), a high-pressure/high-steam wash that cleans all pathogens off.

Every national packer should be using a Chad cabinet and not trying to hand-wash a carcass. Personally, I would not eat beef that came out of a plant that did not have a Chad cabinet. Usually, it's the small, regional packers that don't have one, because the cost is prohibitive.

From the Chad cabinet, the carcass goes into a cooler, which is oddly called the hot box. It's called that because the carcass goes in there hot—it's just gotten out of the steamy Chad cabinet, after all—so it goes in the hot box, where there are now thousands of other carcasses. That's where it stays for about twenty-four hours. The carcass can stay up to thirty-six hours, but it'll start to shrink. As the animal evaporates, as moisture falls off, it's shrinking and losing weight, and the packer doesn't want that because that means less volume of meat to sell.

To prevent that shrinkage, they use what's called a "mister system," which is constantly spraying a fine mist on those carcasses to reduce evaporation. The goal is to keep weight on, cool them down and get them ready for production.

After it has cooled down in the hot box cooler, the side of beef is graded, gets another wash and then goes through a carcass chill on its way out of the cooler and onto what's called the fabrication floor. There, it will get sprayed again and washed again.

Out on the fabrication floor is where it gets separated into primals. We talked about these in Chapter 5, "What Makes a Steak a Steak"—you can look at the diagram on page 8 to see how it's all subdivided. Once that side of beef is moved into the fabrication room, workers are going to take those individual primals apart (into subprimals) and pack them separately, splitting them between the rib and the shortloin. They're going to split the carcass in half at the forequarter and the hindquarter. Have a look at the diagram to see what's in each quarter.

So now we have what the industry calls boxed beef. This is a massive industry, but there is a motto at the meat plants: Keep it cool, keep it clean, keep it moving. This is what keeps you safe.

12

Following the Trail (of Boxed Beef)

J UST LIKE everything else in the industry, the process of getting the meat from the slaughterhouse to the stores is controlled by Big Beef. When I think of "trail" and "cattle," I think of a lonely cowpoke trundling along out on the plains by himself, just his horse and his herd and the big sky above. Maybe he has a harmonica tucked inside his chaps and he'll pull it out later at the campfire he makes after the sun has gone down. But that is as far from the truth as the sun is from Earth. It's a sleepy, gauzy dream. The real-life show is a massive industry tasked with getting the 27.4 billion pounds of meat it produces each year onto trucks and eventually onto your plates.

If the Big Four really did have a hand in designing the specifications of America's long-haul trucks, or even if the Big Four imagines it did, I really can't think of any other industry that would dream of having such an influence on commerce, except perhaps oil. The meat fits in our semitrucks like a hand in a glove, with no room to spare.

Here's a snapshot of how it works:

Big Beef has a system for ground beef, the trimmings, and a system for subprimals. The trimmings get put into large combo bins, which are lined with giant plastic bags, holding two thousand pounds of meat. The bins are put on pallets and placed in the truck. One semitruck can fit twenty pallets, each carrying a two-thousand-pound load of trimmings. If you arrived at forty thousand pounds, your math is right.

The subprimals—your ribeye, your sirloin and so forth—are always trucked separately from the trimmings, and they are shipped as boxed beef, which actually got that name because of the containers they're put in. We sometimes call them breaker boxes, but more often than not, they're referred to as boxed beef. A full truckload of boxed beef will also equal forty thousand pounds. The maximum a semitruck can carry is forty-two thousand. This is the maximum truck cargo weight allowed by the Department of Transportation.

This is valuable cargo. Let's do some quick math to prove it. If I fill a truck full of tenderloins that the butcher or the retailer will in turn sell at $12 a pound, that amounts to $480,000 worth of meat in that truck. That's a mind-blowing amount of money.

Now take that same price for trimmings. Conventional trimmings can be as low as $1.80 a pound. So that truck filled with trimmings might be only $72,000 worth of meat. That's why you're going to load up as much trimmings as you can on a truck to maximize the value—because it costs you just as much money to ship forty thousand pounds of tenderloin as it does to ship forty thousand pounds of trimmings.

That boxed beef and those trimmings are coming straight from the packing house and headed for a distributor. There are thousands of them in this country. They'll buy that truckload and try to sell it as is, or they'll try to sell it to somebody who is going to cut steaks out of it and move it farther on down the chain. Often, the distributor won't even take possession of the meat. They'll sell it to a company like Rastelli Foods in Swedesboro, New Jersey. Rastelli will maximize their profits by maximizing yield, which means they will cut the primals so carefully that they will get as much steak off them as possible, with very little trimmings.

Anyone who is buying boxed beef will keep an eye out for an opportunity to load up on their inventory. If the price of ribeye drops, they'll want to buy low and sell high, whether it's a distributor looking to resell to a retailer, or a retailer looking to buy low and sell high to customers. This is, after all, a commodities market. They will buy those steaks, freeze them, then resell them at the nicer price. The nicer price for *them*, that is.

Boxed beef can be frozen for at least a year, and sometimes is. In fact, you've probably eaten a lot more of that than you'd ever believe possible. You've probably eaten a lot of beef frozen six or eight months and you didn't even know it. You had no clue. There's nothing wrong with it, but it might make it less appealing to know that, so anyone who deals in beef would rather draw your attention away from this fact. No one wants to go to a premier Chicago steakhouse and order sirloin from a stockpile that's been frozen for half a year or more.

Sorry, I didn't mean to ruin your night out, but unless it's farm to table—meaning you know what farm your beef came from and you can practically see it from your table—there is a significant delay between slaughterhouse and sizzling steak.

The trail is the way it is because the packing houses are so highly centralized. From an industry perspective, the method is seen as cost efficient. In their eyes, better to have a centralized operation to oversee rather than hundreds or even thousands of small packing houses all working independently of one another.

All meat is shipped, trucked and moved the same way and cut by the same packing houses. Everything is cookie-cutter. Everything is streamlined.

The question is, how effective is this transport method? Say you live in Florida. There is a good chance the beef you buy at Albertsons in Largo has been shipped from a packing house in Nebraska. Aren't there cattle closer to Florida than the ones being processed 1,600 miles away in Nebraska?

And what happens if the supply chain breaks?

Beef is perishable. Beef is a vital food for life. If there is a problem at one or more of the big packing houses and they have to close, or reduce operations, what happens? What about all that beef? As famed animal expert Temple Grandin warns, "Big is not bad, [but] it is fragile."

The supply chain is made up of many, many steps, and even within those steps, there are a host of substeps. Any time one of the dozens of chains in the overall supply chain—processing, cattle shipping, beef shipping, et cetera—gets bottlenecked for any reason, it can cause a problem down the line. And if you end up with a shortage of meat on the shelves, prices will go up, and people will be left without meat to eat. The point is, there are so many intricate parts to the beef supply chain, and they all have to be managed.

Decades ago, the supply chain was still very diversified. There were small packing plants all over the country, many of them in large cities, processing fewer than one thousand head of cattle a day—sometimes far fewer. Back then, the packers would sell whole carcasses to butchers and retailers. There was no such thing as boxed beef. They didn't cut the primals into subprimals, then further break them down to fit in specially built boxes for big trucks. Meat was never cut at the packing house because there was no room for that. They didn't have the space.

But by the end of the 1970s, the whole industry had transformed, and now nearly all of the processing is done by a few huge packing houses. What we now refer to as "small farmers"—they used to be just farmers—mostly got squeezed out of the picture. We now depend on the food that's being transported in big semitrucks on interstate highways across the country and across the oceans, because we no longer have a variety of local butchers who use local slaughterhouses.

The beef industry does a remarkable job getting beef all over the country, and it has a history of doing so safely. But it is a monolithic operation, and it might be time to consider a more diversified system.

In the meantime, the next time you're zipping down the interstate, salute the meat truck that could be hauling almost half a million dollars' worth of beef.

13

Beef Is Food, but First It's a Currency

LET'S SAY one day you walk into your grocery store, head over to the meat counter and see that the tenderloin is selling for $14 a pound. Maybe two weeks later, you make the same trip to the same grocery store and head over to the same meat counter and see that the tenderloin is now selling for $9 a pound. You look at the package. It's the same brand. You look around at other products in the store, and none of the other prices have dropped. Mayonnaise is still selling for the same price. Cucumbers are still selling for the same price. What gives?

Unlike other livestock, pork and beef are commodities. The market for the cuts goes up and down on a daily basis. There is a morning price and an afternoon price. The USDA publishes a report called the "National Daily Boxed Beef Cutout and Boxed Beef Cuts" twice a day, which gives the price of every primal cut in America. Essentially, this is the wholesale cost of beef cuts in the USA.

In fact, every carcass is tracked every day. Every one of the nearly one hundred thousand head of cattle that are slaughtered is recorded. The USDA tracks whether the animal was a heifer or a steer, whether it graded Choice or Select, how many pounds each cut was and what the weighted average was.

Since the end of World War II, beef has been bosom buddies with the USDA. It is as if the United States Department of Agriculture—which is ostensibly a governing force for all agricultural practices—is really the United States Department of Beef. When a non-meat-industry person was appointed the new head of the Food Safety and Inspection Service in the 1990s, he found the speed dial in his office was set for only two numbers: the American Meat Institute and the National Cattlemen's Beef Association, which are two of the three most powerful beef lobbies in the nation. And nothing has changed since then.

When I buy a new smartphone, it will never be worth what I paid for it again. It will never go up in value. It's the same with my car. But I can freeze beef, and a month later it might be worth more than what I paid for it. In what world can frozen food be worth more than fresh food?

The beef industry has tremendous pull in government. It heavily influences both the lawmaking side and the regulatory side. To you, beef should always be a food, but it's worth remembering it's also a currency that's traded on a market.

What's in a Brand?

AMERICAN GROCERY STORES are as big as oceans. They're huge. If you ever amble down the aisles of a grocery store in Spain, or France, or Germany, or Morocco, or practically anywhere else on the globe, and then walk back into the shivering freeze of a colossal American market, you will know this. They are whales to the rest of the world's minnows, and the proof is in the numbers. The square footage of your average grocery store—your Kroger, your Safeway—is just over forty-two thousand square feet. That's almost an acre of food to buy under one roof. And then there are the warehouse stores, such as Costco, which can be up to two hundred thousand square feet.

That's also not considering that while you're in grocery store A, stores B, C and D are in shouting distance. And E, F and G are around the corner. And all of the shelves in all of the stores are stocked chock-a-block with twenty-five brands each of everything from raisins to ribeyes.

There are more than fifty brands of laundry detergent. More than seventy brands of yogurt. More than twenty-five brands of mayonnaise. Mayonnaise! How many choices of mayonnaise does one country need? And as for beef, there must be thousands of brands. There are nearly as many brands of beef in America as there are stores to sell it.

But it's important for you to know that most of these brands are owned by Big Beef. They create some of the brands in-house as marketing strategies to get more shelf space, and some they purchased from once-independent or family-owned businesses that sold. Niman Ranch is a great example of a company that looks like a small family farm, or at least a consortium of family farms. But they're owned by Perdue, and Perdue is very careful about letting anybody know that. Applegate? Hormel owns it. Coleman Natural? It's a Perdue product. Hans? Draper Valley Farms? Also Perdue.

It's funny to me how people respond to the word "farm." Marketing studies have shown that people are more comfortable buying from "farms." They feel good about buying from a farm. The word "ranch" is good, but it doesn't quite have as warm a connotation. Maybe it seems a bit too commercial. But with a farm, they picture chickens and goats, and maybe a few sheep, all out in a dewy pasture at sunrise.

So what did guys like Cargill and Tyson do when they found out how cozy and cuddly the word "farm" made people feel? They went out and started farm brands. Shady Brook Farms. Shady Brook Farms sounds like a beautiful place. Who wouldn't want to raise their animal in Shady Brook? But it's just a giant Cargill meat and turkey brand that does a great job of making people feel good about themselves.

Your local supermarket, whether it's Safeway, Stop & Shop, Kroger or Piggly Wiggly, sells vast amounts of red meat, thousands of pounds a week. Believe it or not, it's the single largest volume product at nearly every major grocery store. In some cases, it can be 25 percent of the total revenue of a grocery store. So it makes sense that these supermarkets would get in on the action and have their own brands to sell too, which they do. Each and every major grocer in America has a private-label beef brand, which they take a lot of pride in. Safeway's brand is called Rancher's Reserve. Stop & Shop has Nature's Promise. Albertsons has Signature Select. There are dozens and dozens of others.

Yet all of these in-store brands also circle back to Big Beef. You must know this is true, because no one really believes that Whole Foods raises its own cattle. Listen, the meat in Safeway Signature and the meat in Meyer Natural Angus is the same damn meat. Meyer's might be cut a little bit thicker, because they want you to feel you're getting a little bit more of a restaurant-quality steak—because generally the only difference between a store-bought steak and a restaurant steak is the size—but there is an excellent chance that the meat came from JBS, Tyson or Cargill. The steaks might be packaged differently. One might be vacuum-sealed and get a twenty-one-day shelf life, and the other might be in your typical grocery tray with the plastic overwrap around it, which was probably cut in-house and laid out there with a sticker. It arrived at the store vacuum-packed, but the shelf life will now be about five to seven days. But whether it's Safeway's private label or another brand, you can bet that most of them came from the same source. Same meat, different packaging.

Though they are few, there are still private brands out there that compete with Big Beef. But whether it's from the big packers or from an independent label, how can you tell what's what? The question you have to ask yourself, and by that I mean the question you have to ask of the people behind the brands, is how deep into the supply chain does the company really go? How close do they get to the source of cattle? In most cases, not as close as you'd think.

We can take a company like Omaha Steaks, or Allen Brothers in Chicago—or even Certified Angus Beef, which is really just a marketing group masquerading as a beef brand—and ask of each of them: How far into the supply chain do you go? Do you breed cattle? Do you raise cattle?

Say there is a brand claiming to be "fully integrated" or, better yet, "farm to table." From that, you'd think it could be assumed that this company owns ranches and vast amounts of cattle, and that they are deeply involved in the husbandry, rearing and nutritioning of animals. Maybe it could also be assumed that they own a cow-calf ranch for breeding. You feel like you can trust what they're saying because they're this amazing, well-known XYZ Branded Beef Company. But the reality is, most of these beef brands don't own any cattle whatsoever. None at all. They don't buy animals; they don't feed animals. They simply buy beef and put their label on it.

Where do they buy their beef from? They buy it from the big meat packers. JBS. Cargill. Tyson. National Beef. I'm not knocking the packers, I'm just saying they are huge, monolithic companies, and most beef on the market today, despite the vast number of brands stocked on the shelves of our vast grocery stores, comes directly from these packers. This is true whether it's conventional beef or organic beef. That warehouse of choice you thought you had is really only a shoebox.

There's a branded beef company in California that comes to mind. It's a family-owned business that claims to raise a large number of beef cattle. Possibly this is true. But let's put into perspective the number of cattle that would have to be raised in order to sell even forty thousand pounds of beef, which is one semitruck full. It would take approximately 120 cows just to make 85/15 extra lean hamburger trimmings. And that doesn't include the fifteen thousand pounds of middle meats, like ribeyes, striploins and New York strips. That might sound like a lot of steak, but it's only enough to supply one single Costco store for one week. And maybe not even that.

The point is, when a company leads you to believe that all the beef they sell comes directly from their farms, they're kidding themselves. More to the point, they're kidding you. Because once again, let's take a look at the numbers. Say your beef company, Brand X, raises five thousand cattle from birth to slaughter every year and a half. To raise that number of cattle, your company would have to own thousands of acres of grassland. And your company would also have to own a traditional feedlot. So while your company's toiling away raising this one herd every year and a half, JBS is bringing that many cattle to slaughter every single day.

So how can your beef brand compete with a big packer? It can't. What are beef brands selling then, if not beef from their own cattle? If you scratch past the website, and scratch past the marketing, and really get to the company, there's usually not much there. Except for some sophisticated branding and marketing, there's nothing. Most of these independent beef companies are virtual companies with some small office somewhere, with most of their employees working remotely. They usually have a slick website alleging all the things they do in livestock and all the things they believe about sustainable agriculture and humane animal handling. They have images of beautiful, jet-black cattle grazing in pastoral green fields. But guess what? They don't own those cattle. They bought the images from a stock photo site. They don't own a single cow. They are buying the beef from JBS or Cargill, putting their label on it and selling it to you at a higher margin than if you were just to buy your local grocery store's brand.

The way it works at my company, Raise American, is we buy animals at a young age, although we don't always buy the animals, per se. In some cases, we put a deposit on them, so we have some stake in the game with the producer. Let's say I put a $500 deposit on an animal. Now, I've bought the right to buy that animal. I've bought the right to decide what that animal is fed. I've also bought the right to reject the animal if it gets sick or if it doesn't get to the specific weight under the specific feed that I want. In this way, I'm in partnership with that rancher or that farmer. If he gets that animal to the weight I think we will make money on, my company will process that animal, and then the next season, I'll go to back to that rancher and say, "I'll take the next eight hundred head of cattle." So I don't own the land. I don't own the cattle, but I certainly did invest in it. A great way to look at it is I'm a stakeholder—steak-holder!—in that animal.

There are some brands out there that actually do buy cattle. I didn't say *raise* cattle, because that's a very important distinction. They buy cattle, often the day of or the day before the cattle are processed. They do this so they can claim they own cattle, even if they purchased it hours before it was slaughtered. But let's be honest, they're not in the livestock business, they're just brands. They're brokers for Big Beef. Most beef companies have little control of the product their customers are eating.

There are some farmers out there who raise animals just because it's part of their brand image, and this makes no sense to me whatsoever. Maybe this beef company is in Maine, and this small herd they own is really struggling in the conditions, because Maine isn't the greatest place to raise cattle. But because they are a beef brand, they feel they have to have some hand in raising cattle, just so they can say they do. They have nothing but a tiny, token herd. They take care of this small herd of cattle, yet they *still* source the meat they sell from Big Beef.

There are independent brands on the market that have no affiliation to Big Beef, but it's up to you to find them, and it's up to you to ask the questions of them. How long did they own that animal? Twenty-four hours? Forty-eight hours? Or did they buy the animal for the last ninety days, to ensure they didn't get any antibiotics or growth hormones during that period, as their website claims? Ask them, "Do you own your own packing house?" If a company owns their own processing facility, it is a good start. It is also a good indication that they buy their own cattle and do not just broker and relabel products from Big Beef. But you have to ask. Very, very few beef brands own the animals from birth to slaughter, if they ever own them at all.

If you don't want to pick up the phone and call them, and in most cases there is no way to do so, there are other ways to find out where the company sources their beef. To do so, you'll have to cut through the smoke and mirrors they call a website.

The first thing to do is *look at the language*. They use a lot of coded words and phrases, and here are a few to watch out for.

 We partner with: They aren't partnering with anyone. What this really means is "we buy from."

 We source from: Same thing. It means the source of their beef comes from this place. But they rarely have any relationship with any of their cattle producers and probably have never met them in person.

We put together a standard that all of our producers must adhere to: This is a pretty common phrase to paste on a site. Or some version thereof. It makes you feel great, but you've got to understand that it's not likely that anyone from that branded food company is actually going around to any of the feedlots to check any standards at all.

We raise our cattle here: If they can tell you exactly where they keep their cattle (a physical address), this is a good sign. If they can tell you exactly how much cattle they raise and how much they process, even better. You can't raise five hundred head of cattle per year and sell five million pounds of beef.

Please come visit our ranch: If you are being actively invited to an agritourism situation, where a producer wants you to see his or her property and cattle, this is a very good sign.

Meet our farmers: I, for one, think you should take a brand up on this. If there is a producer on their website or packaging, call that office. See if you get a real person. If you do, ask them, "Do you raise cattle for Brand X? How many head do you raise each year?" A legitimate cattle producer would be more than happy to share this information with you.

Second, *look at the package*. By law, every package of beef sold in the United States must have a number listed with the USDA that indicates where the beef was processed. It's called an "establishment" number and it's right there on the label: "EST," followed by a number. Tracking it this way will take about thirty seconds of sleuthing, and all you need to do is plug that number into the interactive Meat, Poultry and Egg Product Inspection Directory on the USDA website. You can find out pretty quickly where it was processed. Or you can search "establishment number 12345" (or whatever), and you'll usually be led to the site. Anyhow, if you look it up and see your Brand X was processed by JBS, you know for sure they're brokers, not beef producers.

The bottom line is, you have a right to know how beefy your beef brand is, and what might just be fluff!

15

What You're Allowed to Say, What You're Not Allowed to Say and What It Really Means

YOUR GRANDMOTHER used to be able to stride into the butcher shop down on the corner and order a pound of ground beef, and that was it. Back then it was probably ground chuck, which was ground right in front of her eyes. She knew it was fresh and she knew where it came from. She didn't have to sort through a staggering number of labels slapped onto the overwrap. She ordered the ground beef and the butcher weighed it, wrapped it in paper, handed it to her, wiped his hands on his meat-stained apron and went on to his next customer.

But you can't buy just a pound of ground beef anymore. What you *can* buy is a pound of all-natural, organic, antibiotic-free, raised with no added hormones, GMO, no-additives, fresh/never frozen, grass-fed, grass-finished Product of America lean ground beef. Oh, and don't forget Prime, Choice or Select. It's enough to make you want to go out and buy your own cow, just so you never have to decipher another sticker.

But what are all the stickers and what do they all mean?

They fall broadly into two categories. You have your "seals" and you have your "claims." Let's start with the seals.

You can think of seals as a "seal of approval," as these are labels that are backed by an organization. It could be the USDA or it could be the Happy Dancing Cattle Clan, but a seal is some organization giving some kind of stamp of approval on your meat. Whether the organization has any merit or not is another matter.

Consider this: the American Angus Association has only one main requirement for cattle to qualify as Angus—the cow must be black. Well, let me correct that. The cow must be mostly black. Hold on, let me correct that further. The cow must be at least 51 percent black. So can a dairy cow, a Holstein, that has more black spots on it than white parts qualify as an Angus under the guidelines of the American Angus Association? Not exactly—black spots on a white cow don't count—but the point is, there does not have to be genetic proof that the cow is Angus. It just has to be mostly black, and it must exhibit some measure of "Angus influence," whatever that means. Maybe you need to interview the cow and find out if it identifies as Angus, who knows.

The Angus breed, more officially known as the Aberdeen Angus, originated in Scotland more than four hundred years ago and was introduced in America in the mid- to late 1800s. It's a very unique-looking cow. If you saw a genetically true

Angus sitting in a pasture among a bunch of other cows, you'd know right away it was a breed apart. Typical characteristics include, of course, the black color, along with a polled head, which is a bony structure that appears like a knot at the top of the head (where the horns would normally be), and a very stocky, very squat body. It must also have what's called a high dressing percentage, which basically means that after it's dead and been stripped of everything that can't be eaten, it must still have a fair amount of weight (also known as meat yield). So a real Angus must be a pretty hefty boy or girl, be as black as coal, be squat and barrel chested and have a knot like a crown on its head.

Unless it's qualifying in America, in which case it only has to be just a tad more than half black in color. That's like me somehow claiming Choctaw tribal rights because I'm 1/57th Choctaw. But there it is. If you have cattle with some black in the hide, you can slap "Angus" on the package and no one has to know that it is not in any way genetically related to the Scottish herd. Angus is now the most common "breed" of cattle in the United States. No wonder, since there's hardly any real qualification. But this beef is called Angus, and it sells for a higher price because of its perceived status as being, forgive the pun, a "cut above."

But here is the caveat. The American Angus Association has created two tiers of Angus. There is the "Angus-influenced," which is the lower tier and the category that the vast majority of "Angus cattle" in this country falls under. Then there is the "Certified Angus Beef." For beef to actually qualify for this label, which is a label issued by the American Angus

Association, the cattle must meet stricter qualifications than just being 51 percent black. They don't necessarily have to be genetically aligned with the ancestral Scottish herd, but there is a far higher standard set for them than the wannabe Angus-influenced cattle.

But most folks don't know there are two tiers. They see "Angus" on the package and they don't realize it's not true American Angus. I mean, come on, if McDonald's, Burger King and Hardee's can sell Angus beef, the bar can't be that high. But it's important to note that none of these chains are selling Certified Angus Beef.

All that being said, there are some seals that do carry weight, and they're worth knowing about:

 The Humane Farm Animal Care is a non-profit outfit started by a woman named Adele Douglass about twenty years ago. This organization issues the **Certified Humane Raised & Handled** seal, which intends to curb animal abuses on the farm and in the slaughterhouse. Seeing this seal should help the consumer be a bit more reassured that employees are trained in animal welfare and handling and that animals are allowed at least a measure of freedom of movement and to engage in their natural behaviors. A big caveat where beef is concerned is that under this seal, beef cattle do not have to be raised entirely on a pasture. So again, consumer beware. But the main credit to this seal is that it is overseen by an outside panel of scientists and veterinarians, and inspections are made annually. Further, it's backed by the ASPCA.

The American Grassfed Association is a non-profit organization that issues the **American Grassfed** seal, and its standards are pretty high. Beef that gets this seal of approval comes from cattle that are fed grass only, no grain ever, and farms are inspected every fifteen months, which is important because inspectors can see the farm during different seasons. Animals are given no antibiotics and no hormones, and no GMOs are allowed. Synthetic pesticides can be used, but the case has to be made for them.

 USDA Organic is probably the strictest government seal, and it really has to be earned. When you see this label, it means the farm where the cattle were raised was inspected annually, and no GMOs, pesticides, antibiotics or growth hormones are permitted. Farms have to be third-party certified to use this seal. Any food carrying this label has to be third-party audited. No ax, no agenda. There is a lot of oversight in this regulation.

Even imported products have to go through the same process to be organic certified by the USDA's third-party group. Who is the third party? Whoever gets qualified by the USDA via the National Organic Program and the National Organic Standards Board. The person should be a valid, credentialed certifier. They're in China, Australia, Uruguay, Brazil. They're all over the world, and they're the ones who give permission to put the USDA Organic seal on the beef, in America or elsewhere. But remember, since the removal of COOL—the Country of Origin Labeling—you would never know you've got a USDA Organic steak that came from Uruguay. You're likely just assuming it came from the United States.

However, there are two grades within this seal, and you need to be familiar with them. If you see **USDA 100% Organic**, you can be sure—whether it's beef you're buying, or granola, or any other product—that every single ingredient that went into the making of that product is organic. If the USDA label does not have "100%" on the seal, the standard to be met is 95 percent organic. That other 5 percent is up for grabs.

 Non-GMO Project Verified is a seal given by a non-profit of the same name. It was started more than a dozen years ago by a small group of natural food sellers, and the standard that has to be met is right there on the label: no GMOs.

These are some of the reliable labels you can look to, but even so, you can already see how redundant they can be. If the GMO issue is covered by the USDA label and the American Grassfed label, you probably don't need your beef to also be certified by the Non-GMO Project Verified label. By definition, all USDA organic is non-GMO. Yet that does not give the extra layer of confirmation that Non-GMO Project Verified does.

Beef companies have to pay for these labels. None of them are free, and none of them are awarded. Providing label claims is a business, not a charity. Ranchers have to pay to have a USDA inspector, called a "certifier," come out and survey the conditions on their farm. They have to pay for the American

Grassfed Association to come inspect. If for some reason they don't pass inspection, they still have to pay. Ranchers have to pay for any certification seal they want on their beef, so you as the customer usually won't see more than one of these stickers on the same package of beef.

But this also raises another question: If the USDA has a stricter code than the American Grassfed Association, why would a farmer choose to go with a less stringent code, however good American Grassfed is, and what does that mean for the beef? It could simply be a case of cost. The inspections are expensive, with USDA NOP (National Organic Program) being the costliest, so perhaps smaller family farms would rather save a bit of money and go with a lower-cost inspection that still gives a decent seal of approval. That's a reasonable choice for a bottom-line farmer to make. But it's still a question worth considering.

However, there are a lot of small organic farmers who don't bother with the cost of obtaining any seals at all, yet their meat might very likely meet the strict code of the USDA NOP, and then some. But these are usually hyper-local farmers who sell to a small community of consumers. If you buy from Farmer Francis up the road, you should have a pretty good idea of the kind of farms he runs. The seals are for the rest of us who buy our beef off the shelves.

So that's what a seal is. A "claim" is a much looser goose, and it's here that you really have to stay awake so you don't get taken in by them. Claims don't need any backing by anyone, and they don't have to meet any standard. They are truth's sidesteppers, and they're everywhere.

I recently came across a product claim on the website of a large organic retail grocer touting its commitment to organic beef: "Like all meat sold at our stores, grass-fed beef must meet our strict quality standards, which require that animals are raised on a vegetarian diet with no antibiotics or added growth hormones." I had to read it a second time, because "vegetarian diet" really caught me up. Cows *are* vegetarians. It's not a lifestyle choice for them. It's not *who* they are, it's *how* they are. They are herbivores, so say their ruminant stomachs, so what's the point of making a product claim like this?

It's an obfuscation of the obvious. This company is willing to bet that when you see "vegetarian," it's going to make you feel like a superior human. Even if you're a human that still eats meat, at least the meat you're eating doesn't. That cow is holy and pure in some way, and that's the cow you're eating. Vegetarian equals healthy, and somehow that means you. Claiming their cows are better because they're fed a veggie diet is like me claiming my dog is better because I provide an environment in which he is encouraged to walk on four legs. Their claim reminds me of the water I've seen that has a "fat-free" claim on the bottle. It's ridiculous!

The worst offenders in my opinion are "all-natural" and "naturally raised." What does that even mean? Was the cow raised by hippies on a commune? Was it homeschooled? As far as the USDA is concerned, "natural" refers to a product that has no artificial ingredients and no preservatives and has been minimally processed. Well, that's easy. Every piece of meat in America qualifies for that. Beef in this country has things added to it—hormones and antibiotics—but neither of those is considered artificial, and there are certainly no pre-servatives. And all fresh beef is minimally processed because processing costs money. No one *maximally* processes fresh beef. So there you have it: all the fresh beef you buy in this country qualifies as natural.

I hope what you are beginning to see is that some beef brands will say just about anything to make you feel good. In fact, we have a name for that in the industry. We call it an "emotional buy."

Recently, I was invited to a ranch in Texas that was selling Non-GMO Project Verified cattle to whomever wanted to buy that beef for their brand. I arrived at the farm, which was a lovely place. But as they were taking me around, I counted only twenty head of cattle. Hmmm, I thought, what's the catch?

The group I was working with had purchased three thousand head of cattle from this very ranch in the last ninety days.

"Where are all the cows?" I asked.

"Well, we buy from other ranchers sometimes…"

I pressed them on it. "Who do you buy from? Can we go see them?"

I got a big fat "no" from them, which didn't surprise me. As you learned in the last chapter, brands are famous for buying from Big Beef and passing the meat off as their own. In this scenario, I, and the group I was with, was being asked by a legitimate national brand to go inspect the claims put on their label at the ranch level. But when we arrived, we saw right away that there were no cows to inspect. Well, except for those twenty. The claims failed even the basic due diligence. This outfit was able to get a Non-GMO Project Verified label without having even a couple of dozen cows offered up for inspection. The worst part of this story is that this is a common occurrence. So oversight is not always what it should be.

Sensing public trust is slipping, the USDA decided in 2020 to propose changes to its existing code that should further strengthen oversight and enforcement of its organic regulations.

In any case, the advice I have for you is to read the claims, sure, but know that most of them are worded to influence you, not inform you. Now you know to beware of the "emotional buy" tactics that are being used.

16

By the Way, What's a Byproduct?

Y OU SEE on packaging everywhere—on vitamins, on skin care products, on soaps—that this product "contains no animal byproducts." But what exactly *is* an animal byproduct?

When it comes to meat, a byproduct is every piece of the animal that is not specifically a muscle cut destined to be steak or hamburger, but is otherwise used in some way. It's *everything* else. Everything from the outer ring of fat, to the bone, to the blood, to the hooves. Do you eat liver? Liver is a byproduct. Might you fancy a little beef tongue? Beef tongue is a byproduct. How about oxtail? Oxtail is a byproduct. Your favorite leather jacket? That's made from hide, a byproduct. Buttons, bandages, cellophane, toothbrushes, dice, piano keys, adhesive tape, shampoo, glue—all made with beef byproducts. Soap, mink oil and crayons are all made with beef byproducts. Sugar? That includes bone char (it's what makes sugar white). That antifreeze you just bought? Beef byproduct. Those tires? Beef byproduct.

What gets tricky is when some of these byproducts end up back in the burgers, and what gets trickier is the packaging language that comes with it.

Let's first start with the process. All the bits of meat, all the scraps that aren't fit for the trimmings pile of which some of your ground beef is composed, ends up in a different kind of pile. Think of these as "super trimmings." These super trimmings come from the meat parts that cling to the bone and the hide and the cartilage. The tough-to-get areas. There might be some veins that get tossed in there, too. None of this stuff gets thrown away. Instead, a machine scrapes it off the hide before the hide goes on to become your leather belt, and scrapes it off the bone before that bone can be milled into material to make your bone china.

Now that you have a nice big pile of "super trimmings," it gets heated, and afterward it's put through a centrifuge, which liquefies the fat, thus separating it from the rest of the trimmings. The fat gets turned into tallow, and what's left is what the USDA and the conventional beef industry think of as lean beef, or what they've come to call "lean finely textured beef." Or LFTB.

The next step in the process for this "lean beef"—this LFTB—is to get squeezed into a tube, where it's exposed to ammonium hydroxide. Why? To remove any bacteria that didn't get wiped out in earlier cleaning of the beef. This is important, because loads of pathogens gather in exactly the places these types of trimmings were extracted from.

Especially the fatty layer that's between the carcass and the hide. In that area, it's like a pathogen singles bar, but that puff of ammonia raises the pH of the meat and destroys any remaining pathogens; at least, that's what it's supposed to do. Anyhow, by the time this carnival of extracted parts comes out the other end of the tube, it looks as creamy as a marshmallow and as pink as a little girl's doll house. How did it turn pink? The ammonia.

This process has been going on for some time. Starting in the early 1990s, this "pink slime" began getting inserted back into things like pre-packaged patties, meatballs and so forth as a filler. The question remains, though: Is it beef? It's a byproduct, because along with the scrapings of meat, bits of collagen, cartilage and the like are also mixed in. But should it be considered beef?

The man who coined the term "pink slime" was USDA microbiologist Gerald Zirnstein, and he claimed it wasn't beef. Twenty years ago, Zirnstein was an accidental whistleblower. Accidental, because he made the comments in an email sent to a colleague back in 2002. But journalists eventually discovered his internal complaints and published them in the *New York Times*. "I do not consider the stuff to be ground beef," he said, "and I consider allowing it in ground beef to be a form of fraudulent labeling."

This byproduct had for decades gone into pet foods and even cooking oil, but Big Beef decided to rebrand it as the pleasant-sounding "lean finely textured beef" and was somehow able to convince the government that not only was LFTB safe to use in ground beef, but that it actually *was* ground beef.

Big Beef and the USDA—the USDA after some wavering—still maintains that LFTB is regular, good old-fashioned ground beef using nothing but modern technology and American ingenuity to use as much meat from the carcass as possible. But forget for a moment the byproducts in it, which in my eyes make it not 100 percent ground beef—I'm with Zirnstein on this—and ask yourself, what about the ammonium hydroxide?

When this filler first started showing up in pre-packaged foods, customers complained about a strong ammonia odor. Who wants to go home on a Friday evening after a long week of work, open up a box of frozen patties (because you need a bite to eat before going out), and be hit with the smell of ammonia? It's nauseating. It's alarming. So Big Beef decided to lower the amount they were using, and guess what happened next? *E. coli* happened.

But to me, the worst part of all this is that you're not being told. You're not being told about the filler, and you're not being told about the ammonia. How could that be? Well, since Big Beef has decided that the filler is not filler, but is 100 percent ground beef, and since they've convinced the Department of Agriculture of this, no labeling is required on the package. Some packers do put "LFTB" on some of their items, but not all of them. And ammonium hydroxide, which in any other case would be considered an ingredient, and therefore listed on the package, has instead been cast as a cleaning agent, and therefore is *not* required on the label.

McDonald's, Burger King and Taco Bell stopped using the filler in 2012, after news reports spurred public outcry. Retailers like Kroger, Safeway, Winn-Dixie and a few others also stopped selling meats that contained it. Note that *ABC News* had to pay an enormous settlement to Big Beef for defamation after their piece on pink slime aired, which might be yet another indication of the power of Big Beef. It reminds me of the CBS *60 Minutes* tobacco debacle back in the mid-1990s, when Philip Morris threatened a lawsuit if CBS aired a segment on Big Tobacco's attempts to hide the effects of nicotine.

The point for you at this stage of the game isn't that the filler is in the ground beef, it's that there are currently no regulations requiring meat to be labeled as such. You're not going to find it in the ground beef you purchase in the meat section, but it will be in the frozen patties, the meatballs—any of the prepared frozen foods that are ubiquitous in American stores. Personally, I'd like to know if I'm eating something that contains low-grade byproducts, or something that's been banned in the EU and Canada and taken off the shelves of several major American retailers.

Incidentally, this kind of filler will also be in any kind of processed meat, and they should disclose it on the label. Bologna. Packaged lunchmeats. And definitely in hot dogs, where they won't likely be beef fillers—LFTB—but they'll be the chicken or pork version of them, for sure. Hot dogs are made from trimmings and they can, and usually do, contain more than one kind of meat. They're often made of a combination of chicken and pork. They might contain other beef products, like cheekmeat. However, the USDA requires these byproducts to be listed on the label—along with all the other ingredients. Conventional hot dogs are high in sodium nitrate, but that'll be listed. They have corn syrup. White vinegar. Dextrose. Sodium lactate. All listed.

Organic hot dogs contain beef, water, sea salt, organic evaporated cane syrup powder, organic cornstarch, organic paprika, organic coriander, organic red pepper, organic white pepper, organic nutmeg, organic onion powder, organic garlic powder, organic mace and organic celery juice. Like their conventional hot dog cousins, it's easy enough to know what's in them, because the ingredients are printed on the package. And there won't be any pink slime.

The point is, whether conventional or organic, the ingredients in a hot dog are right out there for you to see. It's right there on the package. If it's on the label, it's on you to make the decision. But what can you do when it's not on the label? What do you do when filler loaded with byproducts is passed off as ground beef?

The only action you can take to ensure that the food you buy contains no filler, no "lean finely textured beef"—one of my favorite euphemisms of all time—is to look for the USDA Organic label. That's the only way you can be sure that your meat does not contain ammonia-treated filler, or any filler at all, for that matter. When you're out to eat, you're at the mercy of the restaurant, but you can find those places that serve organic, and you'll know you're getting 100 percent beef, with no byproducts.

Organic means no byproducts. And it definitely means no ammonia.

17

A Change in the Beef World

BEEF IS beef, right? Cows will always be cows, and we'll always like to eat them. Who among us can remember a time when steak or meatballs or meatloaf or pot roast—or, for God's sake, hamburger—was not a staple on our table? At most dinner tables in this country there will be some kind of beef served a few times a week, even if it's incorporated into a side dish or mixed in with a sauce. But we don't just wait for dinner. These days, we often eat beef three times a day. I think the birth of fast food pretty much sealed our love for eating beef all day. We swing by the drive-thru for a taco or a burger, we pack a lunch of leftover beef stew, or we stop by that Tex-Mex place near the office and get a beef fajita. If not there, the corned beef at the deli. And of course there are the die-hards, who will probably indeed die hard, who eat steak with their eggs for breakfast. Beef is to us what rice is to Asia. Think about it. Think about how many times beef has been in your diet in the last week. It's probably even more than you realize. But our environment cannot sustain this level of consumption, at least not the way the conventional beef system currently functions.

When I was growing up, we might have had steak once a week, and it was considered a real treat. The steak was non-grade sirloin, tough as shoe leather, but it was what my father could afford on a carpenter's wages, and we didn't know any better, so we ate it and we liked it. The point is, we didn't eat beef so casually. Eating steak was special. And it sure wasn't a twenty-ounce steak. I mean, some of us can remember when McDonald's came out with the Quarter Pounder. We were tripping. A quarter pound of beef? Are you kidding me? That sounded like a lot. Do you know how much it is? It's four ounces. That's it. But it sounded like a lot because it was a lot then. We just weren't used to eating that much beef that much of the time.

Eventually, people started to eat meat at every meal. Sausage in the morning, a pulled pork sandwich for lunch, and maybe a hamburger or a steak on the grill for dinner. It stayed that way for a while. For one thing, meat is very inexpensive in this country. For another thing, Big Beef has done everything it can to lure you into eating more meat.

Consumers are speaking up now. They want healthier beef, healthier alternatives to beef and, above all, a healthy planet. Despite its omnipotence, Big Beef is hearing their voices for the first time in its history. As a result, there are a lot of innovations out there that are giving the conventional rancher a run for his money.

But before we look at what's new, we need to look at what's wrong, and some of what's wrong is the way we farm.

Corn was once the salvation of American farmers. It was the cowboy of crops that swooped in and brought cattle ranching back from its post-war brink. And in the great American tradition, more was better, right? More corn fed more cattle; and much more corn fed much more cattle, which meant much more beef and, most of all, much more money. At least for the fat-cat packers. What could possibly go wrong?

A lot, it turns out.

Livestock farming and fossil fuels are two leading causes of the rise in methane gas. The *Guardian* reported in July 2020 that in the last twenty years, the release of methane into the environment has risen more than fifty million tons a year, and a lot of this is from collective cow belches. Cow bellies don't take kindly to corn because it makes them very gassy, and the end result is atmosphere-eating methane that is, quite literally, a major contributing factor to climate change.

There are almost one hundred million cows in the United States at any given time. This is an incredible number, considering how many are slaughtered each day. The number of cows worldwide? One and a half billion. According to the USDA, a beef cow in the United States can eat a ton of corn if it is raised on a feedlot. That doesn't include the silage it will eat, which is a mix of fermented corn and greens. Remember, this is what's fed to a *single cow*. Multiply this by one hundred million, and you get what? My calculator just imploded, but I know that you get one hundred million ruminant stomachs trying to process something they can't, so one hundred million cows contributing unnecessary methane gas into the atmosphere all day, every day. Year upon year, decade upon decade. It's a funny thought, until you realize how sobering it is. And just for the record, it's the belching that releases the gas, not the tail end. It's their burps, not their farts, that are wreaking havoc.

Methane is an exceedingly harmful greenhouse gas, one that manages to very effectively trap heat—thirty times more effectively than its closest competitor, carbon dioxide. Have you ever been in a sweltering attic on a summer day? There are no windows and the heat gets trapped. The temperature soars. That's kind of like what methane does to us.

"Animal farming and fossil fuels have driven global emissions of the potent greenhouse gas methane to the highest level on record," reported Jonathan Watts for the *Guardian* in July 2020, "putting the world on track for dangerously increased heat levels of 3°C to 4°C."

One answer to this problem is grass-fed. Grass-fed cattle burp a whole lot less than corn-fed cattle do. Some will argue that because it takes more time and land to raise them, they're a methane menace. But there are now phenomenal natural supplements that are great methane reducers (I go into this in greater detail in the last chapter, "Final Thoughts: Lively's Perfect World"). Yes grass-fed beef costs more, but it doesn't cost us in the same way greenhouse gases do.

Let's get in the wayback machine again: In the 1970s, the United States began to make the switch from leaded to unleaded gasoline. This was a mandate by the federal government, when the scary truth about lead poisoning could no longer be ignored. We weren't drinking the gasoline, of course, but we were inhaling its exhaust fumes, and that put highly toxic levels of lead into our bloodstreams. With so many cars on the road, and with people caught in bumper-to-bumper traffic six out of seven days a week, lead was in every single breath we took. Unleaded gasoline was introduced in 1974. Did it cost consumers more? Yes, it did. Yet in twenty years, we had completely eliminated leaded gas in automobiles in this country.

It was part of a larger effort to clean up the air—Richard Nixon (yes, a Republican) passed the Clean Air Act in 1970—and we can see that the legislation was effective, because we can *see*. If you question what I mean by this, look at a photo of Los Angeles in the seventies, and you'll get what I'm saying. There was so much smog, it's insane. People were walking around the city like zombies because they could hardly see two feet in front of them. So our lungs got cleaner with the reduction of pollution, and our blood got cleaner without all that lead mucking it up.

The federal government moved to eliminate leaded gasoline as part of the Clean Air Act, but it has not led the charge when it comes to reducing methane. That mantle was taken up by everyday Americans. More and more beef consumers started looking for alternatives to conventional beef, and the demand for organic took root. And to give credit where it's due, the market responded. After organic began to take off, the call came for grass-fed beef, and the market responded as well. But as the environmental crisis deepens, some are rethinking the way we farm livestock.

There's good reason for that. Corn is as bad for the soil as it is for the cattle, at least in the way it's grown as cattle feed.

The corn we grow to feed our cattle is usually a monocrop—grown year after year on the same land. At best, it is a duocrop, alternating years with another seed, like soy or wheat.

Many farmers tend to prefer monocropping or duocropping, and that makes sense. They are producing something that they know is in high demand. They can focus on one thing—growing corn—and do it well. They can arm themselves with the pesticides and herbicides they know they'll need—and they *will* need them. Overall, it's a relatively safe venture financially, and without a lot of surprises. And overall, it's terrible for the soil.

Why? For one thing, monocropping attracts pests like nothing you've ever seen. If I'm a pest who loves corn and I find a two-thousand-acre farm full of it, I'm going to tell all my friends about it and we're all going to come and feast on it. And if I discover it growing there the next year, I'll be back the next year and the year after that, or at least my DNA will be programmed to inform my descendants to come back year after year. Monocrops are meal tickets for pests. They may as well just get cut a welfare check. They don't have to work at all to find food. They can just sit back and know it's going to be handed to them. Except, of course, when they eventually die from the toxic chemicals designed to eradicate them.

Monocropping also robs the soil of nutrients it needs to thrive, mostly nitrogen. All of the good stuff gets sucked out of the soil without being replenished the way it would if there were some type of rotation in place. It becomes sick soil, and sick soil can't produce healthy plants. What does the farmer do to compensate? Fertilize it. So the answer is more chemicals. By the way, keep in mind that the chemical company Monsanto—now owned by Bayer—was/is a big player in the corn seed business.

What it boils down to is this: corn-fed cattle harm our air, and the corn itself harms our earth. The way we raise cattle is harmful; there's no question. None at all. The silver lining of all this, though, is that a lot of innovation has come out of trying to heal the environment. One of the more interesting is biodynamic farming.

Apricot Lane Farms in Moorpark, California, became famous when the documentary *The Biggest Little Farm* debuted in 2018. The film follows a young, middle-class white couple as they give up the urban grind for the rural grind. The husband, John Chester, is both filmmaker and farmer on this project, and he shows us through soft lens and vivid colors what it is to create and inhabit what seems to be nothing less than Shangri-La. Before our very eyes, the Chesters create a harmonious and profitable farm, where we come to find out that coyotes are just misunderstood and that a big, lovable pig can make it through any health crisis if she is loved well and loved abundantly, particularly by a rooster. Okay, it was a good flick, and I was glad the pig lived. I could have done without all the hyperbole, but the main point of it was to show that biodynamic farming is a viable way forward.

But what is biodynamic farming? It started in Austria one hundred years ago. Austrian philosopher and spiritualist Rudolf Steiner is claimed to be the Father of Biodynamics, and the practice is essentially an exceedingly holistic approach to farming. The principal theory is that the farm itself is a living organism and, as such, each aspect of that farm is an integral part of it—from the farmer, to the pigs, to the goats, to the cows, to the plants, to the insects. If one is out of balance, all are out of balance. Steiner was concerned about the degradation of food, as farms were becoming more mechanized and pesticides and fertilizers were being introduced. His answer was, as with many things, a return to old ways.

Today there are more than 350,000 acres of biodynamic farms in nearly fifty countries. The non-profit Demeter Association is the certifying body in the United States. It reports the growth of biodynamic farms in this country to be at about 15 percent each year, based on how many farms apply for accreditation. Many people consider organic farming an outgrowth of biodynamics, and I don't necessarily think they're wrong about that. It's likely only a matter of time before we see a wellspring of biodynamic farms popping up.

In the meantime, there are also alternatives to conventional beef consumption arriving front and center, and that includes blended meats.

Blended meats are just what they sound like: meat blended with something else—maybe some spinach and falafel. Or maybe it's a beef blend with mushrooms and peas. A lot of the people who go for blended meats we call flexitarians—they want beef, just less of it. Let's face it, some of us can afford to be flexitarians some of the time. In any case, watch for many more blended meats in the near future. They won't just be on the grocery shelf, but they'll also be popping up more often on menus, too.

Now let's move on to lab meat, which sounds really gross, so most people like to call it "cultured" meat. This is also pretty much what it sounds like: meat that is grown from a stem cell, specifically to produce food, not to clone an entire animal. It begins with the removal of stem cells from the cow. The cells are put in a petri dish with some amino acids and carbohydrates, which is what helps them grow. After a while, voila, you have grown a steak. It's a no-brainer to see that the effect on the environment is far less than the effect conventional cattle have on the planet. According to a joint study carried out by the University of Oxford and the University of Amsterdam, cultured meat could in theory generate 96 percent *less* greenhouse gas than conventional beef. That's mind-blowing to me.

In theory at least, lab meat should be safer to eat as well, since it won't be susceptible to all the diseases cows are exposed to on the feedlots, nor subject to the extensive handling. The beef processes are very clean and very well regulated in America, but zero chance is better than a slim chance.

Lab meat is closer to reality than you might think. A lot of startups have bought into it, and you can expect to see some products hit the shelves in 2022, so be on the lookout.

Of course, you already know about plant-based meats. Studies show that although they are less harmful to the environment than conventional beef, they still cause greenhouse gases. Regardless, are they healthy? Chris Kresser, bestselling author of *The Paleo Cure*, says no. Kresser cites a report obtained through the Freedom of Information Act that indicates one of the key ingredients in the Impossible Burger—one of two plant-based meats currently available—is SLH, a soy-based protein additive that provides meat-like taste and color. This bioengineered additive does not meet the FDA standard, and, what's more, Impossible Burger put the product on the market without admitting to the FDA that it had not done adequate safety testing! This doesn't mean SLH is bad, but it means the FDA cannot determine if it's fit for human consumption. Yet, Impossible Burgers are on the shelves.

Beyond Burger is the companion to Impossible Burger, although it is partly derived from a pea protein isolate, not soy. Like the Impossible Burger, this meat substitute has a remarkable number of ingredients that I wouldn't necessarily say are good for you. And from a flavor profile and good old-fashioned contentment, I'll stick with my cow patties.

Regardless of whether it's lab meat, biodynamic farming or other innovations in the pipeline, it's clear the beef industry will have to take critical strides to improve its position in today's hyper-focused area of climate change.

18

When a Sixteen-Ounce Steak Is Not a Sixteen-Ounce Steak, and Other Lies

LAST SUMMER, a guy I know cornered me at a barbeque to tell me about the best steak he'd ever had. "Oh my God!" he told me. "It was three inches thick!"

Um, since when did the thickness of the steak ever have anything to do with how good it is? It's ridiculous what some people's perception of a good piece of meat is. So you're telling me I can take a nine-year-old dairy cow that's so old she can barely walk, club her in the head and cut a three-inch steak out of her and you're gonna love it? That's the dumbest thing I've ever heard. But it's all part of the mixed-up mindset of beef eaters, who have been told what they should like by the beef industry for so long, they may not have actually stopped to consider what tastes good to them.

Let's be clear. There's no more flavor in a three-inch steak than there is in a one-and-a-half-inch steak, just like there's no more flavor in a foot-long hot dog than there is in a six-inch hot dog. There's more hot dog, but there's not more flavor.

Here's something else: fat doesn't always add flavor. The IMF, the traces of intramuscular fat that creates the marbling, absolutely does add flavor. But the ring of fat hugging the outside of the steak? That does not add flavor. That fat is separated from the meat by a thick, impermeable membrane, which means there is no way that belt of fat can seep through, jump across or crawl under that membrane to flavor your steak. It's impossible. It can't happen. If you put a fatty piece of meat on a grill, all that fat does is drip down and then light up like an inferno. That's not flavor, that's flame. I mean, you could really take the time to trim the fat, render that fat really slowly in a cast iron skillet and then cook the steak in that rendered beef fat, and you'd have a ton of added flavor. That would be phenomenal. But who's doing that? We're not Gordon Ramsay here. (And by the way, while we're talking fat, if that fat ring around the steak is yellow, that's a good indication the steak is from an old cow.)

Yet, how much are you paying for that belt of fat, just to have it burn up right in front of you? You may as well be burning money. But you still buy it. The butchers pre-cut their steaks and showcase them in the meat counter, so that as you pass by it your eye catches on a beautiful red-and-white sixteen-ounce ribeye. My mouth is watering just thinking about it. But let's take a closer look at that ribeye. There is probably an inch of fat on it, which will weigh somewhere around four ounces. So now you're down to a twelve-ounce steak. Yet you're being asked to pay for a sixteen-ounce steak. You'll pay for that sixteen-ounce steak, but you won't get sixteen ounces. Instead, you'll get twelve ounces of meat and four ounces of nothing.

Here's another exaggeration: bone-in. There's no way in hell the flavor on a bone permeates the meat. If anything, it works the other way around and the meat flavors the bone, so the only good news there is for Fido.

When a restaurant charges you for a twenty-ounce tomahawk steak, you're only getting about ten ounces of meat, because you can bet that half of the weight is the huge dinosaur bone they left on there. Does the bone add flavor? No, not a bit. You can do things with bone that create a flavor profile, like render it and make a bone broth. That's a great use of the bone. The marrow has great uses as well. You know, when I see somebody at a restaurant with bone marrow cooked in garlic, that's awesome. That's great. Now you're getting flavor from the bone. That matters. But when I see a giant bone-in steak, I think, what the hell? The only value that bone has is aesthetic, and the only value in that is an Instagram selfie of you posing with it like you're Fred Flintstone.

Not long ago, I saw a giant bone-in filet mignon. It was a ten-ounce filet, and I'm positive the bone was half the weight. You can't eat it. You can't digest it. Maybe it made the person who ordered it feel cool. Maybe they thought it looked great on the plate. But it did not add to the eating experience or the flavor of that meat.

I'd always recommend, especially at a restaurant, staying away from the bone-in product, unless you want to get a porterhouse or a bone-in ribeye just because you're sentimental and a traditionalist, and it brings you back to the days when

Dad ordered it. If you're value shopping and you want to get more meat for your dollar, the bone-in product is more Instagram than anything else.

The next red flag is Kobe beef. Author Larry Olmsted exposed the Kobe sham a few years back, first in some articles he wrote for *Forbes*, then in his book *Real Food/Fake Food*. What he revealed was that all of the Kobe beef promoted on menus across America was *not* Kobe at all, which makes sense, because the only item rarer than Kobe beef is the Hope Diamond. It is so rare that it represents less than 0.2 percent of the beef consumed in Japan. Most Japanese have never had the opportunity to eat Kobe beef, even though Kobe is a Japanese product. When they have had the chance, they've had to dig deep into their pockets, because it costs more than $200 a pound. So does it make sense that in Japan, where it is produced, it is so rare that hardly anyone has had it, but you, all the way over in America, could hop on over to your neighborhood Fuddruckers and get some? Of course not. But Fuddruckers had it on the menu. I don't have a problem with Fuddruckers. Hell, my first job in high school was manning the grill at a Fuddruckers in Ventura, California. But they're Fuddruckers, for God's sake.

Back in 2015, approximately fifteen pounds of Kobe beef, on average, was being imported to the United States each day, which was somewhere in the neighborhood of four hundred to five hundred pounds a month. By 2019, that number had increased to an average of about thirty pounds a day (eight hundred to a thousand pounds per month). Yet, think about it. That's thirty pounds of Kobe beef a day for an entire country. There is so little Kobe beef produced that each beef product is assigned a ten-digit number, so the beef can be traced back to the very cow it came from. Each and every one has a verifiable lineage.

Olmsted called Kobe beef in American restaurants "food's biggest scam," pointing to the laughable fact that until 2010, Japanese beef wasn't even allowed into the US market, yet this didn't stop restaurants from claiming Kobe all over their menus, anyway. It was faux Kobe and they knew it, but their customers did not. In 2014, a class-action lawsuit against a number of offenders attempted to stop the fraud. The few restaurants that serve this Japanese delicacy must now have a license from the Kobe Beef Marketing & Distribution Promotion Association to prevent the faux Kobe, and there is an expensive and rigorous application process.

What makes this deception even more insidious is how expensive even the fake Kobe beef is. A 2016 investigation by *Inside Edition* noted that so-called Kobe beef sold for as much as $55 an ounce back then. Three-Michelin-star restaurant Le Bernardin in New York City reportedly charged $110 for what it advertised as Kobe beef. But when asked to show the Kobe beef certification by *Inside Edition*, the manager vanished, much like the credibility of many steakhouses, including the renowned Old Homestead Steakhouse. It charged between $175 and $350 for what the Kobe Beef Association identified as bogus Kobe beef. When pressed on the matter, the owner responded, "You're getting hung up on what the name is." So if you sell me a Ferrari 250 GTO that turns out to be a knockoff made by Volkswagen, am I getting hung up on a name?

Why is Kobe so exclusive? The cows that give us Kobe beef originate from a very isolated, mountainous part of the country. Because of that isolation, and because of feeding trends that varied from the norm even up through the centuries—a thousand years ago they were draft animals used in rice production—the taste of the beef from these cows has always been very distinctive. And rumors of their coddling turn out to be true. These cows are often fed beer and wine, and even given massages, all in an attempt to keep them happy and relaxed. The pastures they're raised on sound like veritable cow spas, but the thinking goes that the more relaxed the cow is, the less stress it has and the better beef it makes.

The ironic truth is that the few Americans who have had a taste of real Kobe probably think it's awful. It was not meant for the American palate, or the American way of consuming food, which is in larger portions than the Japanese. Taking a bite of Kobe is like eating a large spoonful of butter. I can't think of anything more disgusting, unless it's cod liver oil. But tell us it's exclusive, and we want a piece of the action. Tell us it's exclusive *and* available everywhere, *and* at a reduced rate, and it's clear we've suddenly lost all cognitive reasoning. But it hits our special button (this beef is rare), our comfort button (Fuddruckers is my Friday night place) and our savvy button (it's only $25!). It's being sold to us on three emotional fronts, *emotional buys*, so we check our reasoning at the door and buy in.

There's something else that really bugs me, and it involves Wagyu beef. Wagyu beef isn't even a "thing." In Japanese, *wagyu* means "Japanese cow." Wagyu isn't a specific cattle breed but could be cattle from four choice breeds that are raised under specific, very rigid protocols, at least in Japan. Kobe, for example, is considered Wagyu beef.

But what about Wagyu that's raised in America? (Yes, there is American Japanese beef, if you can believe it.) The qualifying factors that Japan established get muddied to the point that American Wagyu, such as it is, can be half Angus, or even more than half Angus. American Wagyu is watered-down Wagyu.

In any case, how can you verify that a steak is really Wagyu, American or otherwise? As far as I can tell, a restaurant can claim Wagyu on the menu without having to back up the claim. Determining for yourself whether it is or it isn't would take detective-like knowledge of steak that most people don't have. It will be well marbled, but what else? Even I would be hard-pressed to pick out a genuine Wagyu steak based on what it looks like. This is why dodgy butchers and restaurateurs feel free to put a high price on fakes and pass them off as the real thing.

There's one more piece of fiction I'd like to get off my chest, and that's how the restaurant manages your food when you order your meat medium rare.

Medium-rare beef has to reach an internal temperature of 135°F "resting," which means sitting on a plate with no heat or cover. Chefs consider this the ideal temperature for a flavorful and tender steak, but not every chef hits that target. People make mistakes, kitchens get busy, orders get backed up, and if the chef overcooks a steak and the customer sends it back, an expensive cut of meat has been wasted. It gets dumped in the trash. But when has a restaurant ever wanted to foot the bill for a mistake? Never. So what tends to happen? Chefs will undercook the steak on purpose. The customer orders medium rare and gets a raw cut of beef back. If the customer doesn't complain, great. If the customer does complain, the meat gets tossed back on the grill and comes back medium rare. As far as the restaurant is concerned, that's better than having to toss it out altogether.

There are other ways steakhouses trick out their meat. Not high-quality enough? Slather it in butter. This might be tasty, but it just means all the goodness is coming from the butter and not the meat. As I noted in an earlier chapter, they may also label old steak "dry aged," which in this case means "dry" and "aged," and you should run from it. They've also been known to use MSG or other additives to tenderize meat that is otherwise tough; that is, meat that's past its prime.

The diminishing quality of steakhouse beef is not a new problem. Even in the mid-1990s, food writers were lamenting the decline of American beef due to lax grading standards. Beef's waning popularity at that time made it expensive to produce top-quality meat, so the USDA began grading it on a curve. Today, some steakhouses still milk their subprime beef for all it's worth, while taking a prime cut of your wallet.

Don't forget, your server in these high-end restaurants is basically a classy, well-trained salesperson. He or she is there to maximize your check for the restaurant's cash register and their tip. They know as much about the beef as they know about the salmon or the lemon chicken, which is usually next to nothing.

So now you know, and now your eyes have been opened. Don't pay for extras that don't offer anything extra, and if you see Kobe sliders on the menu, say something.

19

The Cuts You Probably Don't Know About (but Should)

HERE ARE a lot of cuts out there that you've probably never even heard of but that make for really great eating. These are the cuts that hardly ever make the *final cut*, pardon the pun, to actually become a steak, and end up getting ground into hamburger instead. It's a shame, because really good meat is not being fully valued for the flavor it can offer.

The ribeye, the porterhouse, the filet mignon—that's what the packers like to sell. All the steaks you see featured on the menu at your favorite restaurant or the ones sold to you to toss on your grill are easily available because those steaks are relatively quick and easy to cut from the carcass. They're pretty sizable, at that. This means big profit with little effort.

Conversely, something like the chuck, which is taken from the low shoulder of the animal, is somewhat more difficult to cut. It also has a lot of bones in it and doesn't yield all that much meat. It can have a lot of nice marbling, but as shoulder meat, it has a lot of gristle, so because of that and other strikes against it, poor chuck usually gets tossed in with the trimmings.

Look at it this way. If I'm the owner of a big packing house, pretty much my only concern is the highest yield possible at the swiftest speed possible. I already know that nothing is going to waste on the animal. Every bit of the trimmings will end up as ground beef or in hot dogs or hell, even dog food, so I don't care about that. So why should I bother to take extra time and care, spend more money and resources, to give you a $4 chuck steak on special at Costco, when I can spend zero extra time and zero extra resources, and just give you that same chuck for $1 less as ground beef? For the love of profits and yield, it would make no sense.

We're lucky, though, because there are some beef processors who see value in these pieces. They save chuck from the trimmings floor, and much more.

Let's take a look at some of the underappreciated cuts of beef you should keep an eye out for.

Chuckeye steak. Much of this shoulder cut is only good for ground beef. Or it might also end up in stew. You can make a delicious stew out of chuck. Or a pot roast, all of which I mentioned in an earlier chapter. It's the shoulder of the cow, so it will have a lot of tough, gristly meat because of all the connective tissue. Once that gristle and toughness is cut away, though, you're still left with a sizable amount of meat, from which a chuckeye steak can be cut. You can also cut part of it into a blade steak, also known as a bottom chuck steak, which comes from under the shoulder. The blade steak is going to be more tender than the chuckeye.

Anytime you're dealing with chuck, it's imperative that the butcher cuts it with the grain, meaning the direction of the muscle—you can see it like you can see the grain of a piece of wood. If it's cut with the grain, it can make as good a steak as any out there. If it's cut against the grain, it'll be tough as hell. Just like wood, if it's cut with the grain, it's smooth; if it's cut against the grain, it's rough.

Flat iron steak. This is also cut from the chuck. This is the "top blade" cut, opposite the blade steak. It is highly marbled and tender. It's usually cut about one inch thick.

Absolutely nothing was known about this cut until about twenty years ago, when some beef marketers went on a full-out campaign to educate chefs and stores about how great it was, at the same time convincing beef processors it was worth the time and effort to cut this meat into steaks. It took several years, but if you're seeing flat iron steak at your grocery store now, that's why.

Hanger steak. This used to be known as a butcher's steak, because it's the cut most butchers liked to keep for themselves, and there's good reason for that. It is a very, very flavorful piece of meat. It's at the round end of the loin and is wonderfully tender. It's becoming more and more common to see hanger steaks, but that didn't use to be the case.

Flank steak. This cut comes from the belly of the cow. It can be very tasty, but very tough if not prepared well. It is very lean; there's hardly any marbling, so it's probably among the healthiest cuts you can get, and among the most affordable. It's also known as a jiffy steak in some parts, and you may have heard of it as a London broil.

Skirt steak. This steak also comes from the belly. There is the outside skirt, which is the diaphragm muscle, and the inside skirt, which is the transverse abdominal muscle. This comes from the beef plate of the cow, which is the upper chest, directly below the ribs. This steak has a very beefy flavor, and if you marinate it, the meat will absorb those flavors well. It's why fajitas can be so good, because skirt steak is often used in fajitas.

Flap steak. This is what the *San Francisco Chronicle* once called "the little underdog of the beef world." Flap comes off the bottom sirloin. It's tucked above the flank. You remove the flank, take away the fat layers and there is the flap. It must be thinly cut across the grain. If not, it will be too chewy. You'll feel like you're chewing meat-flavored Hubba Bubba. But if it's cut right, it is most definitely a steak worth getting to know. This is probably my favorite of the lesser knowns, and I'm lucky enough to have a local butcher who routinely brings in flap meat for me.

Tri-tip steak. This cut comes from the bottom of the sirloin. I don't know why this steak is as economical as it is, because it comes as well marbled and is as packed with flavor as any rib-eye. Tri-tips are great for grilling. If you want to try your hand at kebabs, tri-tips are ideal. Tri-tip steak is very popular on the West Coast, primarily in the Bay Area, but not as popular on the East Coast. But ask for it, and your butcher can find it.

Petite tenderloin. This is also a part of the shoulder, but it's farther out from the shoulder. It's the teres major muscle, and you can tell by its name that it is tender. It's one of the most tender cuts on the whole animal. It cooks, acts and eats like a filet mignon. If you cook it right, it will reward you. I think cutting it into medallions is a good idea. I sear mine and leave it pretty rare in the middle. I really enjoy that steak, but it's just not out there. Yet it's a really budget-friendly cut of meat. If you can get a butcher to cut it, you're in for a treat. I've cooked it for friends, and they're like, "What *is* this?" But you're probably not going to see it out. You'll have to ask for it.

Shank steak. Also known as beef shank, this is where we get beef osso buco from. It's a steak cut from the leg and it's relatively thick. It's incredibly flavorful, but it's not something you're going to see everywhere. It's a chef's preparation. You've got to know what you're doing. It's not like making a pot roast.

Sirloin caps. In Brazil they're called *picanha* and are popular in Brazilian barbeque. This cut comes from the tip of the top sirloin.

Ribeye caps. These cuts come from the top of the ribeye. These steaks are extremely tender and will be pricey. From this, you'll also get the ribeye filet, which is a thick, lean steak. It differs from the ribeye itself because it's thicker, but it weighs the same.

You're going to see a little more of cuts like flank and skirt on the shelves. If the packer thinks they can get more money for them, or even a hanger steak or a tri-tip, then they'll pull it off the animal, process it and put it out on the market. But typically, they don't get much more than ground beef out of any of it. It can be hard to find some of the mid-tier cuts of meat, which are good eating at a low cost. Mostly, you'll find them at specialty butchers.

I'd encourage you to try any and all of these. They're gaining in popularity, but most of these cuts are still budget-friendly enough for you to buy them and experiment with them. You can buy enough flap steak to screw up a few times without feeling like you're throwing your money away. So buy the flap steak and experiment. Buy the tri-tips and try them on the grill. Ask your butcher what cuts he likes that don't bust the bank, then take them home to your kitchen. Pour yourself a bourbon, roll up your sleeves, put on your playlist and start to experiment. See what works.

20

Butcher the Butcher with Questions

MY GUESS is that most Americans have never encountered a real butcher. People buy their meat where they buy the rest of their groceries, which is at an arena-sized national chain store, plodding through the aisles pushing a grocery cart the size of a Honda. Few people shop on Main Street anymore, because there is no Main Street anymore, and few people go to the butcher shop, which is now crammed between the dry cleaner's and the 7-11. They pass it fifteen times a week but never take notice, because they think they get everything they need over at the Piggly Wiggly. Stop for a moment and think where your town's butcher shops are located. Points for you if you know. If you don't, you're among the ranks of many.

Let me tell you something. The guy you see behind the meat counter at your Kroger or your Winn-Dixie or your Piggly Wiggly? He's more than likely not a butcher. There are still butchers at grocery chains, but most likely they're meat managers, and they won't be dealing with customers very much. The guy who most customers see is not a butcher. This guy will be sporting a bloodstained apron, but he's not a butcher. Chances are he's been brought over from produce or bakery. He might be called a butcher, but he's really just a meat handler. (I say "he," because, sadly, less than 25 percent of meat handlers in this country are women, and the percentage of actual butchers is far, far less.)

His main priority is to keep the meat counter stocked, slice your ham and grind your beef. That's it. He's a twenty-year-old college kid on a summer job, and maybe he'll stay on for a while, because the pay is better than what he'd get as a bagger and the benefits are good. But if you ask him about beef, he won't know what to tell you. Maybe the label on the cut of beef you want to buy says Kobe, but you've heard how rare Kobe is, so you ask him, "Is this really Kobe?" Yup, he'll say, and walk away, because he really does not know if it's Kobe or dairy cow or chuck, and he really will not lose sleep over the answer he gives you. He was told to put the label on the package, he did it and his job is done.

A true butcher learns a craft. They know meat like a Nantucket fisherman knows fish. It takes a long apprenticeship to learn how to handle a side of beef, how to move it without damaging it, how to break it into primals with finesse. And how to manage yield to maximize the value of the meat. It's enough of an art form that there is a Butcher's Guild and a prestigious World Butchers' Challenge every year. A quality butcher will have often been raised on a farm and come to the work that way, or will have trained at fine institutes, like the Culinary Institute of America, or through programs offered by the James Beard Foundation and the like. Does it surprise you that universities offer certificates in meat cutting? They most certainly do.

But you have to keep in mind that not every butcher is a master butcher. It's up to you to ask questions to find out what kind of butcher you're dealing with. The better the butcher, the better the beef.

So where do you begin your search? As I've said, the least skilled meat guys are the ones in your grocery store. Don't bother asking them anything. They pretty much know as much as you do at that point. Not that they're not smart, nice people; they're just not skilled in the art of meat cutting. If you ask them the hard questions, you'll be putting them on the spot, forcing them to make something up or toe the company line.

So maybe you ask around, you ask your neighbors, maybe you go on social media, and after a bit, you've got some recommendations for some good butcher shops. What do you do next? You go into the butcher shop and you ask questions. Because you need to know for yourself what kind of meat he's dealing in. Here are some questions you can ask.

Was the animal humanely raised and humanely processed? You have to get into what's behind the beef before you get into anything else. Why? Because it's the single most critical factor in quality beef. You might have the juiciest-looking steak sitting right in front of you, but if it wasn't humanely raised, do you really want to eat it? Because as we know, the animal who is treated poorly gives poor meat. Inhumane treatment, which includes being crammed onto crowded feedlots and pumped full of antibiotics and hormones, creates highly stressed cattle. And this is *bad* for you. So you need to find out if there is a strong humane animal welfare standard for the meat the butcher buys. And what is his definition of humanely raised and humanely processed, anyway? Find that out.

How does he know? Let's say the butcher says, "Yes, all the beef I purchase is humanely raised and humanely processed." Can he prove that? A good butcher will be happy to prove it. Many butchers have visited the farms or ranches they buy from, and they're proud of this part of their job. They can tell you which farm they bought it from, what that farm's standards are and why they buy from this particular farm. Their answer can also tell you a lot about the relationships they have formed with their local or state agricultural communities.

If the beef's not local, why not? There could be a very good reason. Maybe the cattle in your area are not fed what he thinks they should be fed. Maybe you live in Vermont, and the long cold winters and dry summers mean the cow has to eat too much dried-out grass and has to forage too much. Or maybe the butcher wanted a particular certification that no local farmers could provide. Ask the questions and listen to the answers.

Did he cut this primal himself? In most cases, the butcher will buy a primal, but not always. Sometimes they're buying pre-cut steaks, and pre-cut steaks are a dead giveaway that they're buying from the Big Four packers.

Another way of finding out if they're Big Four buyers is to say, "Hey, listen, can I get that cut into a one-inch steak?" If they tell you they can't do that, well, then you know right there that they aren't cutting their own steaks. They don't even have the equipment. They're buying pre-cut steaks and putting them on the shelf like a typical retailer. If they're cutting their own steaks off the primal they bought, they'll pull that steak out, cut it for you and bring it right back to you. If they aren't, you know they probably aren't any better off than the meat handler at Winn-Dixie.

I've pissed off a lot of butchers this way because they know I'm calling them out. I know they're just buying conventional meat from a big commercial packer and calling it whatever they want. And these places aren't cheap. So if I'm going to get a Cargill product, I may as well go to Winn-Dixie and buy it for half the price this snooty gourmet butcher shop is selling it for.

I can't completely fault these guys. There's a demographic that will believe anything that makes them feel good. And as long as these shops aren't changing any of the label claims that come on the proverbial "boxed beef" they're selling, technically they aren't doing anything wrong.

How and where was it aged? Some butchers will throw out a claim that their meat is aged, but they won't give away anything else. So you dig a little more: "Was it dry aged or wet aged?" Maybe they say dry aged. "Where?" Uh, where we bought it from. Well, what does that even mean?

You need to ask them specifically what they mean by this claim. If the butcher says he dry aged the beef himself, I'd ask to see the dry-aging room. It's not a small thing—you have to have a very large space. So you ask, "Can I see it?" If a butcher shop has a dry-aging chamber, they will be all too happy to show it to you. Thrilled, even.

What about your ground beef? The butcher may or may not source his ground beef from the same place he gets his other meat, and some of that ground beef may qualify as what's known as "forced meat"—highly pureed or ground products, the main ingredient of which is meat, but with other garnishes mixed in with it. Some butchers stock a lot of forced meat, so it's always a good idea to ask!

Watch what they're doing as they're packaging your meat. I've watched some people as they're buying their meat. They'll say, "Please trim the fat; I don't want that much fat on there," which is a perfectly reasonable request. Like I said before, why should you pay for four ounces of extra fat that isn't going to be used? But you have to watch the butcher. He will weigh the steak, price the steak, he'll even pull the tag off the scale— he'll pull it off and stick it to the counter—then he'll trim the fat off, wrap it up and put that same price right back on, very carefully right in front of you. In this case, you have to specifically say, "No, I don't want to buy that extra three inches of fat. If you trim it off and then weigh it and price it, I'll take it."

Can you show me the box? This is the most important question you can ask your butcher if you're in doubt about the claims they're making about their beef. The box is like the steak's birth certificate. It's the butcher BS detector. Everything you need to know is on that box.

Whatever you're looking for—whether it's Choice, Prime, Wagyu, Angus, organic, grass-fed—the box will tell the real story, as required by the USDA. Let's say the steak you want to buy is marked Prime but it doesn't look prime at all. It's hardly marbled. You ask the butcher (or summer intern!), "Hey, is this really Prime?" He mumbles yes. "Well, can I see the box?" You can do this anywhere they sell meat—at the grocery store or at the butcher shop, any meat handler who's any good will be more than happy to show you that box.

Recently I walked into the Edgartown, Massachusetts, Stop & Shop, and I saw some Prime steaks. I believe they were Prime New York strips, and they looked pretty good; I'd say the marbling was there. But the price didn't seem right for Prime. If I remember correctly, they were selling for $9.99 a pound. It sounded too good to be true.

So I asked the guy, "Is this Prime?"

The guy pointed to the sticker on the tray with the over-wrap on it, which of course said, "Prime."

"Would you mind showing me the box?" I asked.

He smirked and rolled his eyes, but he went in the back and came out smiling with a big white box with "USDA Prime" stamped on it. I asked him to show me the primal, and it indeed was what it said it was.

"Why the price?" I asked.

"They're on special. That's what we do."

I bought them and they were phenomenal. They tasted just like I would have expected them to taste if I'd eaten them in a restaurant.

If you're dealing with a highly knowledgeable butcher, you shouldn't be afraid to ask questions. Never be afraid to even share what you're doing. I mean, let's say I'm having a party tonight and I'm grilling for ten people. I should be able to go to my butcher and ask, "What do you think?" I should be able to discuss everything with him, from portion size to the vibe I want to have at the party. He might ask, "Do you want to put on a big show and grill some amazing things, or do you want to have something more low-key?" You have a conversation, and he offers you a range of options based on what you're trying to achieve. This is the kind of relationship you want to build with your butcher. You want a meat mentor.

The bottom line is, the guy at the meat counter is there to sell meat. Lots of it. So he's making claims to charge you as much as he can for that meat. Your job is to make sure he can substantiate those claims. You don't need to make this an interrogation. And maybe it's not something you want to do on a busy Saturday, with a line of customers behind you. That's just being confrontational. It's not a contest, and you're not there to embarrass this guy. But if you go in when it's quieter or agree with the butcher on a good time to come back, he should be happy to have this conversation with you. Or, if you're at the grocery store, the meat handler will bring in the store's meat manager. That person will be more knowledgeable than anyone at the meat counter, no question.

My hope is that you find a really nice local butcher shop that has a lot of understanding about where their meat comes from, that they're highly selective about where they source their product and that they've done a lot of due diligence and research, and maybe even visited some farms and ranches. A butcher doesn't have to be high priced to be high quality, and they don't have to have a degree from the Culinary Institute. They don't have to have a degree in anything at all. They just need to know all about their meat, including where it was sourced. And if you're armed with the right questions, you will find the right butcher.

21

Opinions Are Like Oxtails— Every Cow's Got One

WHY WE still call it an oxtail, and not a cow tail or a bull tail, I don't know. But an oxtail is an oxtail, and God slapped it onto the ass of every cow. And just like every cow has one, every asshole has an opinion. If you don't believe me, just stand near a backyard grill on a Saturday afternoon. You'll hear more bullshit there than you'll hear anywhere else in the world. Who knows, maybe that's how we got the word "bullshit" in the first place—a bunch of idiots were standing around a flame bragging about how much they knew about beef. Let me tell you something: most people know zero when it comes to what makes a good steak, but that hasn't stopped them from being assholes who think they invented it.

Let's start with the oxtail itself, a cut most of the backyard posers would never even think of eating. They've probably never even heard of oxtail. If they saw it on a menu, they'd skip right past it and go straight for the striploin. But it's one of the most flavorful pieces of meat you'll find. Basically, it's the tender tissue between the butthole and the tail. It only weighs around two pounds and it's normally cut into two-inch lengths. Because of the marrow and collagen mixed in with the meat, a deeply rich flavor emerges when it is slow cooked. And oh, is it tender. We don't really see too much oxtail for sale in this country. A few pieces are removed from the animal on the fabrication floor at the same time the internals are removed, and oxtail is one of them. It's not really profitable to sell—a retailer can only get a couple of bucks for it—but because it's such a tasty part, quick-handed workers will often pocket them. A packing house that kills a thousand animals a day will wind up with only seven hundred oxtails. Well, they've got three hundred employees. You do the math.

So why am I telling you about the oxtail? Because most people, when they hear what it is, won't eat it. They'll stick to what they know—or what they think they know, because the absolute truth is, a lot of beef eaters don't know the first thing about beef, and they definitely don't know anything about what makes flavor. They think they do, but they don't. Their opinions are so big, they could set up house under them: "This three-inch steak is incredible! I only get the porterhouse from O'Malley's. Did you see the bone on that tomahawk? It was phenomenal!" I've heard more blowhards spewing more bullshit than one man should have to endure in one lifetime.

But what *does* affect flavor? There are probably sixteen answers to that question. It's like asking someone how to raise a good kid. You can't say it comes down to one thing, right?

Because there are too many variables, from luck to love, and it's nearly the same with beef.

From an industry standpoint, there are a few primary indicators that are going to affect flavor, and the first of these is genetics. Each breed is predisposed to certain characteristics. Some are predisposed for tenderness, some for size, some for fat, some for flavor.

You take the Piedmontese, a breed out of Italy, and you take the American Angus—the certified one—and they're each genetically predisposed for different qualities. The Piedmontese is unique because of a genetic mutation that makes it "double muscled." The beef doesn't have a lot of marbling, but it is very tender and lean, thanks to that gene fault. The Angus, however, is bred for marbling. It's the fat that makes it tasty.

After genetics, we look at age. How old was the animal? A twenty-four-month-old cow is going to taste vastly different than a thirty-six-month-old. As cattle age, the flavor changes. An older cow could have a beefier flavor, generally speaking.

Now, what did you feed that cow? Let's assume it was grass-fed. Okay, but what was the condition of the grass? If I'm feeding an animal in northeast Missouri, where it's humid and gets a fair amount of rain and the grass is lovely, and then I'm feeding another animal in eastern Oregon, where it's high desert, there's isn't much rain and the animal is really having to forage, the beef from these two animals is going to taste different. And if I've fed one in a feedlot and the other in a pasture, that will affect the flavor, as well.

These are all nuances that add or detract from a flavor profile. But you can't isolate one.

Next, was it dry aged or wet aged? We've already had a good look at the kind of difference that makes.

So far, we have genetics, the age of the animal, what it was fed, how it was fed and how the beef was aged. Now let's look at stress. Years ago, Temple Grandin conducted a study on how stress on livestock affects meat quality. She looked at cattle, pigs and sheep prior to slaughter, and studied both psychological and physical stressors, including weather, the fasting some of them have to tolerate, the stress of transit to the slaughterhouse, and fighting among the animals, which is more likely to happen in close quarters. On the hours-long drive to the slaughterhouse, and then in the holding pen, the animals are mixed with other animals who are strangers to them, and this can cause them angst.

All of these factors produced stress in the animals, but the most detrimental to the beef that came off these animals were the psychological stressors. A lot of lactic acid is produced in this state of acute stress, which leads to a lower pH and an overall tougher meat. If an animal is generally a relaxed animal throughout its life, and humanely processed—which includes being stunned properly before it is killed—the same animal will be a much better eating experience.

So now we have genetics, age, what it's fed, how it's fed, how it's aged and stress levels that can affect flavor. Now let's look at this from another angle. Let's just say all things are equal, and you and I were sitting there with beef from the same cow and the same cut of meat. Let's say it's USDA Choice, and let's go with ribeye. And we decided we were each going to cook one, then I was going to eat your steak and you were going to eat mine. Or we'd eat half of our own steak, then trade. Your steak would taste vastly different from my steak, just based on who cooked it.

You might cook yours a little longer; you might salt and pepper yours more; you might use olive oil and I might use butter. You might grill yours; I might broil mine. *Who* cooked it and *how* it was cooked can change the flavor profile so much it's almost baffling. I mean, a really talented steak chef could take an okay piece of meat and knock your socks off. Blow you away. And someone who's not a great cook can take an amazing piece of meat and destroy it. Char it. Screw it up. Just decimate the flavor.

I know this guy in LA, he's a great chef. He cooks a bone-in porterhouse bone side down, the strip straight up, like a tee-pee. When I saw him doing it, I told him it was insane because the bone doesn't add any flavor. You know where I fall on that. But he had a trick up his sleeve and knowledge on his side. This is what distinguishes him as a master chef. He was using the bone to heat up the meat. If you've ever cooked a T-bone, you probably just dropped it on the grill, and when you started to cut the thing, you got near the bone and the meat there was super rare. I mean, not even rare, but pretty raw. At some points it's so uncooked it won't even come away from the bone, right?

But this chef knew that if he heated that bone up, it would get to a point where it was actually cooking the beef from the inside out. He was using the bone almost like it was an oven, an extra heat source. It got so hot, it was able to cook the meat closest to the bone really slowly and gently. The bone heats up really fast, but it doesn't really burn, so it was a brilliant idea. After he was finished, he let the steak come back to room temperature, then he slowly seared it on one side, and then he slowly seared it on the other side. He took an hour to cook this giant, twenty-four-ounce, bone-in porterhouse, but it was phenomenal. I could never do that. I don't have the skills, the patience or the knowledge. So to me it was just a beautiful, beautiful thing to see this guy work his magic.

But the point is, you and I would have a vastly different experience with that steak. Even two cooks of equal skill will produce different results. Professionally prepared, backyard prepared or novice prepared, it's all going to taste different. Some people like to sear it on the grill. My favorite is to sear and then bake: you put the whole tenderloin on the grill until you get this great browning on the outside of it, then you put it in the oven for a slow cook. It's beautiful. The British do that a lot, but now the trend is to reverse sear it, which is when you cook it in the oven first before finishing it on the grill.

All that's going to affect the flavor. Not just a little bit. Drastically.

The final variable is you. What mood were you in when you ate the steak? Were you sitting at a restaurant alone drinking a glass of wine in deep meditation? Were you at a party having a great time? "God, this steak is so good!" Maybe it was just okay but your mood was off the charts, and that affects flavor. The steak you thought was so great was probably just some freaking local Stop & Shop Choice piece of whatever, but you were having a good time, and whoever cooked it used butter and salt, and that crap just tastes good. You remember that steak as one of the best steaks you ever had. So you go back to the steakhouse and get the same steak, but this time it's just so-so. You're disappointed, but you didn't consider that it was just the overall experience that was so fantastic the first time.

It works the other way, too. I mean, I've gone into a steakhouse by myself when I was in the worst kind of mood. I'd had a terrible day and I thought what I really needed was a steak and a martini before I went home. And you know what? It was awful. I mean, it wasn't my favorite steakhouse to begin with, but I went in with a bias because I was in a crappy mood. The martini came and it was kind of warm, not chilled like I like it. When the steak came and it was slightly overcooked, I was like, "Screw this place." But if we change the scene a little bit, and you put me in there with two buddies and a couple of hot women, then it's a totally different experience. "This steak tastes great! This martini is wonderful!"

So what can you do to zero in on a good flavor profile for the beef you prepare?

You can do what the standout restaurants do, which is develop consistency. Take your cue from the great steakhouses, like Mastro's in Scottsdale and Peter Luger's in Brooklyn, which have mastered the science of cooking what their clientele likes. I can walk into Mastro's and know I'm going to get a great steak nearly every time, no matter what mood I'm in.

How do you do that in your own kitchen? I think you have to explore and experiment until you find what you like and not be afraid to try new things (like oxtail!). Don't listen to the asshole at the cookout who has plenty of opinions that he's all too happy to share. Instead, try the flank, the brisket, the flat iron, the flap meat. Grill it, broil it, butter it. Do whatever to it, until you come up with a process that works for you. Then once you come up with a system, stick with it.

When I tell people to try new cuts, as well as new ways of cooking their meat, what I'm really saying is, get to know steak. Get to know steak like a sommelier gets to know wine. I always think of this older guy I met a while back. He was a really nice guy, a very successful electrical engineer, and we were out one time at a place that I would never order steak from. It was more like a Chicago pub kind of place. It was a small neighborhood joint, and those places just don't move a lot of volume, so I'm always wondering how long the meat has been there. How talented is the chef who is cooking this New York strip? I think about these things. Pubs like that don't spend a lot of money on steaks because they don't move a lot of steaks, so it's the kind of place where I might get a burger, or wings, or a chicken salad, but not a steak. I don't want to watch them screw it up and I don't want to be disappointed.

But he ordered this giant New York striploin. It came to the table, and I could see right away it was a Select piece of crap, no marble, burned, charcoaled on the outside, and the ends were curled up, which meant it had sat on the grill too long.

"Do you want to try it?" he asked.

"No."

"You sure?"

"No, I'm good, thanks."

He didn't say much, but at the end I asked him how it was. "Ohhh, you missed a good steak. You missed a great steak."

Then he told me he only eats steak three or four times a year. So how the hell would he know what's good? He hardly ever eats steak, so how would he be able to tell if it was great or not? It's like asking a teenager about vintage wine. Again, nice, kind, successful guy, but not a beef aficionado. He didn't know enough about beef to know what he was truly missing.

I think, like anything we decide to do in life—tennis, golf, chess—cooking a good steak takes practice, but the more often you do it, the better you'll be at it. Are you familiar with the ten-thousand-hours rule that Malcolm Gladwell made famous? It suggests that anyone who practices for ten thousand hours, talented or not, can master the skill they are working on.

Don't worry, I'm not suggesting that you quit your job and ditch your family in search of creating the perfect steak, but that what Nana and Gramps said turns out to be true. No, not that your face will stick that way, but that practice makes perfect.

If you're afraid of messing up, the first thing you need to do is stop being afraid. So maybe you don't go out and buy the $46 ribeye from the uptown butcher. Maybe you buy a $16 ribeye and practice with that. Because look at it this way: if you can make a $16 Choice ribeye taste great, imagine what you can do with that Prime cut!

Branch out from that filet mignon you've always reached for, which is the world's easiest cut to cook. It's as easy to cook as a hot dog. There's hardly any effort at all in a filet mignon— the cow did all the work for you. So try different cuts. Work on it. I call it "time with the tools." Try it on the grill. Try it in the cast iron skillet. Try it in the oven. Find the method and the cut that you are most happy with. Then focus on it, write it down and continue to develop your consistency.

One of my favorite things to do in the world is on Thursday night, when I come home alone. I'm a single dad and I don't have the kids on Thursday evening. So I'll get home around four o'clock, after I've picked up a New York strip from Stop & Shop (it could be organic grass-fed, but if they're out of that, I'll grab something else). I'll come home and grill it up, medium. I'll caramelize some onions right on my stove and pour them directly onto the steak, and that's it. I have the steak and onions, and I'll sit back with a bourbon, maybe smoke a cigar out on the deck, hop into the Jacuzzi, watch some crap TV, fall asleep, and then the next day I'm ready to go. Some protein and a little time off are all I need. No one telling me what to do or what has to be done. Everyone's got their therapy, and that's mine. Once I do all that, I'm in bed by ten p.m., up by six a.m., and I'm Superdad till Monday.

With that indulgent downtime, that meditation time, that focus, I've become so good at making the New York strip that I don't even have to think about it. I know exactly how many minutes on each side, I know how to brown the onions without burning them and I can do it all with my eyes closed. That's my go-to thing. You'll eventually have your go-to thing. And it will be whatever the hell you want it to be.

What will happen naturally is that the more you experiment, the more you start to appreciate what part of the animal it came from and then where the animal itself came from. You'll come to know its attributes and the best practices for preparing it. You'll stop looking for an off-the-shelf answer and start creating results for yourself. And best of all, you'll shape your own opinions about what you like, and you can forget about what anyone else tries to tell you.

The bottom line is, discover what you like. If you want a beer-fed, back-massaged, boneless Kobe steak for $170, go for it. If you want a pan-seared, butter-basted ribeye, go for that. Or maybe a grass-finished tenderloin from the grill. It doesn't matter—just learn what you like. This is not dinner with your dad at Sizzler anymore. There's a lot out there just waiting for you to sink your fork into it.

Final Thoughts
Lively's Perfect World

I AM NOT sure if I was destined for this business, but I do actually stay awake at night thinking about things like this, things like what a perfect cattle world would look like. I think about what the best cows would be for the industry and for the consumer. I think they would probably be Aberdeen Angus or Hereford, because I believe they are hearty and genetically superior animals. I think about the pastures they'd be raised on, which would be vast green ones in the ideal climate of a place like Missouri, or even southeastern Ohio. I think about what they'd be finished on, which would be some of the finest feeds in the world, from flax to milo/ sorghum to alfalfa hay. The cattle would have slow, relaxing, leisurely days in the sun, and after two and a half years, they would be processed into amazingly tasty, extremely healthy beef products.

This is what I think of at night. In the light of day, I'm a realist who knows that the perfect cattle and the perfect field and the perfect climate and the perfect atmosphere can't be whipped into existence when you're talking about feeding the masses every day in a country of three hundred and thirty million people.

But that realist knows the industry can be better and can do better. That industry can serve us better. It can halt, or even reverse, the damage factory farms are doing to our environment. The realist in me knows that a simple push in one direction or another could make a massive difference.

Bear in mind, I don't think the problem lies solely on the shoulders of the Big Four packers. The amount of consumption in this country is through the roof, and it's not just the Big Four shoving it in our faces. It's us lining up with our plates out in front of us, salivating for more. In essence, you could say we are no better than the cattle at the trough, eating everything that comes off the wagon. They give it to us, we eat it and we stick around for more. If people don't think or don't care about what they're eating—where it's from, who processed it, how it got on their plates, how it was prepared—then why should the industry care? People are buying it, and that's what matters to them.

I would also say that most people I personally know in Big Beef are decent, hardworking people who truly care about putting out safe, quality beef products. There just hasn't been much emphasis on the sustainable side.

Yet, there is hope, because the packers are starting to wake up, and a good example of that is grass-fed organic beef.

Several years ago, people began to call for healthier food, and they especially began to call for beef from cattle that were humanely treated. More and more consumers began asking for it, and the industry responded. Grass-fed went from small, hyper-local farms to an industry-wide phenomenon that is rapidly growing. For the first time, people are telling Big Beef what they want instead of the other way around.

Maybe now it's time to demand even more. There's a lot of talk about sustainability as a benchmark the industry should try to reach. But I think that could be too little, too late. According to the United Nations Food and Agriculture Organization, if we keep on this path, the world has less than sixty years of food production left. Their figure is based on the current rate of soil erosion, which to a great extent is caused by environmentally unsound farming practices. So that means we have about sixty more harvests left. Ever. That's chilling.

Doing better means going regenerative. We need farming that revives the land and removes greenhouse gases.

What would that look like? Can my lofty idea of a small, idyllic farm, with cattle being gently raised on green pastures and alfalfa hay, overlap with the reality of large feed facilities? Can Big Beef address the environmental crisis and still feed the masses?

I believe it can. Big Beef can start by taking lessons from the regenerative farmers already out there doing the work. In Chapter 17, I covered biodynamic farming, which definitely sits under the regenerative tent. But in general, any farmer who is focused on soil health and repairing the decades of damage caused by conventional practices is a regenerative farmer. As many of them like to say, "It's not the cow, it's the how," a great phrase if I ever heard one, coined by Bobby Gill, a leader in the regenerative movement.

One farmer I know who gets the "how" right is Lindsay Klaunig, owner of Trouvaille Farm in Athens, Ohio. Klaunig practices "prescriptive grazing," which uses animals as tools to improve the land. Her farm is on an Appalachian plateau, a place of hills and hollers in what used to be coal country (and is now surrounded by natural gas wells and propane pipelines). The acreage is on a steep incline, making it especially susceptible to erosion. But Klaunig thought it was ideal for regenerative farming. "What can you do on a grassy, thirty-degree slope? There's nothing appropriate you can do, so we're making food on that slope," says Klaunig. "How else can you do that without causing erosion, except grazing animals? When you perennially graze animals and you do it responsibly, there are always roots in the ground, which hold the soil and prevents erosion."

When animals aren't managed properly and graze to the point that the pasture looks like a desert, the overgrazing doesn't just cause erosion, it causes greenhouse gases. Plants are what get the carbon out of the air—through photosynthesis—and stored in the soil. If there are no plants, the carbon dioxide is in the air, where it becomes a greenhouse gas. And greenhouse gases trap heat. Hello, climate change.

What Klaunig does, and others like her, is maximize carbon sequestration. She grazes her animals on a tight rotation, so they never graze too hard and compromise the land.

There's far more to regenerative farming than this, but what I'm saying is that I think regenerative farms like the one Klaunig runs are not just the way of the future, but the way of now. And I wholly agree with Bobby Gill, who believes livestock aren't the problem, but the solution. We don't need to get rid of livestock; we need to use livestock to generate a healthy planet.

"You can use a hammer to build a house, or you can use a hammer to knock someone upside the head," Gill said in a TED Talk that's gone viral. "It depends on how you use the tool. The same thing goes for livestock. You can mismanage livestock on your land and totally destroy that ecosystem. Or, you can properly manage your livestock and regenerate the health of that ecosystem."

Another area of focus in my "perfect world" is feed.

We know now that corn is the accidental devil here. The crops have ravaged our land, and the methane it causes is destroying our atmosphere. We need to change the feed, and one option I like is clover. Studies in the United Kingdom have shown that cattle eating a mixture of white clover and grass tend to have the smallest methane release. Clover is a legume, and this is ideal because legumes have this fantastic trick they do: they capture nitrogen in the air and return it to the soil. It's a natural fertilizer. So the clover/grass mix is, in many ways, a win-win situation: less methane in the air, more nitrogen in the soil.

Seaweed is another option, and an even better one than clover. As great as clover is, it takes a long time to grow. But seaweed grows rapidly. In the right conditions, it will see about six inches of growth in a single day. It also doesn't need fertilizer. It doesn't need to be watered. Pests hate it. And tests show that cattle do exceedingly well on seaweed.

One test in Australia, in which freeze-dried seaweed, a variety known as *Asparagopsis*, was fed to cattle as a supplement, had such promising results that the scientists observing the data thought their equipment was broken.

Adding seaweed to cattle feed can reduce methane emissions by 80 percent. It won't affect flavor because it's not the primary diet, it's a supplement. I'd like to see it cultivated, harvested and pelletized, then fed to the cattle in their general feed ration.

There are other feed options being explored, but clover and seaweed are two of my favorites.

In addition to improving the feed, there are a few other ideas I have that I've been wanting to get off my chest for a while now:

- We have the ability to genetically crossbreed cattle that not only gain fast, and, therefore, are more efficient on their daily average gain, but are also predisposed to produce less methane.

- We need to entice more agricultural students into the science of raising cattle in best practices. Agricultural programs across the country are not growing; they are limited to four or five very good universities. If universities would invest time and energy into the sustainability of commercial farming, we'd all be far better for it. Unfortunately, most university sustainability programs are focused on forestry or urban planning, and we need more sustainability programs focused on agriculture.

- Cattle should be raised closer to the processing plants so that there's less transport involved in getting the animal to the place where it will be slaughtered. Animals are currently being forced to spend up to ten hours in transit, which is a huge waste of fuel and labor. It's also quite stressful for the cattle—some would say inhumane—and a stressed animal reduces the quality of the beef.

- We can use even more of the cow than we already are. Big Beef in the last twenty years has really come around in offering us more cuts at greater value. But what about the oxtail? What about the tongue? The cheekmeat? These are very edible, and sometimes delicious, parts of the cow, but average consumers don't see value in them, so the packers do not always use them the way they could.

Our beef supply chain is far from perfect, but all in all it has made great strides in the last decade or so to get cleaner, better and truly more humane. The USDA does a phenomenal job protecting the millions of pounds of beef going through our food supply chain each day. Keep it cool, keep it clean, keep it moving—it is that standard that keeps the quality in the beef you eat.

My goal in writing this book has been to inform you. I want you to know what I know. The next time you buy that pound of ground beef, I want you to be able to think about how it ended up at your local meat counter. The next time you buy that steak, I want you to feel comfortable that you have a pretty good idea what that cow ate, where it was processed and even the monumental effort it took to get it to you. I want you to feel comfortable enough now to walk into a local butcher and talk beef with him. I want you to feel ready to try a few cuts you haven't tried before and a few new cooking methods that may seem foreign to you.

Be well. Respect the animal and the people who prepared it for you.

Think about your options. And just as you would with wine or cheese, or any other epicurean enticements, eat what you like, not what someone else says you should like, and never be afraid to try something different. Even oxtail!

For the love of beef!

SCOTT LIVELY

Acknowledgments

I TRULY WANT to thank the following people who have been so influential in the creation of this book, whether it was as a significant influence on my experience in the world of beef or actual direct involvement in the creation of *For the Love of Beef*. This book would not have been accomplished without a long cast of characters influencing me positively, negatively or simply subconsciously.

First of all, Patti McCracken, thank you for your patience, time, research and honesty. Most of all, thank you for sticking with me to see this book through to the end. No one would be reading this book on beef if it were not for you. You are an amazing writer and have become a great friend.

Now for the rest of you Kings, Clowns and Contributors, who may or may not have known about your contribution to this book. This list is in the order in which I encountered you along my timeline in the beef world, and not in order of any significance:

Tim Turner, Joel Rissman, Matt Grove, Issac Wiesenfeld, Randy Perry, Dave Dawson, Bala Kironde, Bob Meyer, Mel Coleman Jr., Doug Holbrook, Bob Huskey, Tyson Apperson, Kevin Smith, Jared Peterreins, Heather Gilmore, Patrick Sangursky, Ray Rastelli, Tim Donmoyer, Randy Bobe, Charles Bradbury, Marc Broccoli, Kent Haeger and Nicholas Tarpoff.

A special thank-you to Roman Kettler and Mike Skubisz of Mastro's Steakhouse in Scottsdale for making me fall in love with steak all over again, and for treating my family like their own. And thank you to Joey, the steakhouse waiter in Boston who knew as much about beef as I know about nuclear fusion; thanks to a local butcher who tried to tell me flap meat and top sirloin were the same thing; and finally, thanks to anyone and everyone who loves food, mostly a perfectly prepared cut of beef.

Notes

Introduction

And as a $111 billion-a-year industry: "Statistics & Information," USDA Economic Research Service, ers.usda.gov/topics/animal-products/cattle-beef/statistics-information.aspx.

The average American eats: John Misachi, "How Much Meat Do Americans Eat?" World Atlas, September 26, 2018, worldatlas.com/articles/meat-consumption-in-america.html.

Surprisingly, only 5 percent: Zach Hrynowski, "What Percentage of Americans Are Vegetarian?" Gallup, September 27, 2019, news.gallup.com/poll/267074/percentage-americans-vegetarian.aspx.

2: Why Your Beef Ain't COOL

Nearly 80 percent of the organic beef: "Back to Grass: The Market Potential for U.S. Grassfed Beef," Stone Barns Center for Food & Agriculture, April 2017, stonebarnscenter.org/wp-content/uploads/2017/10/Grassfed_Full_v2.pdf.

Most of that beef is from cattle: "A Review of U.S. Tariff Rate Quotas for Beef Imports," USDA Foreign Agricultural Service, April 25, 2016, fas.usda.gov/sites/default/files/2016-04/2016-04_iatr_beef_trq.pdf.

According to Inc. *magazine*: Peter Economy, "McDonald's Just Made a Stunning Announcement That Will Completely Change the Future

of Fast Food," *Inc.*, January 17, 2018, inc.com/peter-economy/
mcdonalds-just-made-a-stunning-announcement-that-will-
completely-change-future-of-fast-food.html.

4: What's Prime and Who Decides?

The beef grading system originated more than a hundred years ago:
Sources for How Beef Makes the Grade infographic: USDA (usda.
gov) and study.com.

7: What Should the Cow You're Eating Be Eating?

All that good grass eating: "Grass-Fed Beef: Is It Good for You?" Nourish
by WebMD, September 30, 2020, webmd.com/diet/grass-fed-beef-
good-for-you#1.

8: What's Good about Your Beef?

One of the items on its current list: USDA, "Dietary Guidelines for Americans 2020–2025," dietaryguidelines.gov/sites/default/files/2020-12/
Dietary_Guidelines_for_Americans_2020-2025.pdf.

9: What's Bad about Your Beef?

Then there are the big feedlots: "Sector at a Glance," USDA Economic
Research Service, ers.usda.gov/topics/animal-products/cattle-beef/
sector-at-a-glance.

Both the Johns Hopkins Bloomberg School of Public Health: Pew
Charitable Trusts and Johns Hopkins Bloomberg School of Public
Health, "Putting Meat on the Table: Industrial Farm Animal
Production in America" (report of the Pew Commission on
Industrial Farm Animal Production, 2008), pcifapia.org/_images/
PCIFAPFin.pdf.

More than thirty-four million pounds: Maryn McKenna, "After Years
of Debate, the FDA Finally Curtails Antibiotic Use in Livestock,"
Newsweek, January 13, 2017, newsweek.com/after-years-debate-
fda-curtails-antibiotic-use-livestock-542428.

"Bacterial resistance," the report stated: As cited in Maureen Ogle,
"Riots, Rage, and Resistance: A Brief History of How Antibiotics
Arrived on the Farm," *Scientific American* blog, September 3, 2013,
blogs.scientificamerican.com/guest-blog/riots-rage-and-resistance-
a-brief-history-of-how-antibiotics-arrived-on-the-farm.

12: Following the Trail (of Boxed Beef)

As famed animal expert: Temple Grandin, "Big Meat Supply Chains Are Fragile," *Forbes*, May 3, 2020, forbes.com/sites/templegrandin/ 2020/05/03/temple-grandin-big-meat-supply-chains-are-fragile.

14: What's in a Brand?

The square footage of your average: "Supermarket Facts," FMI (The Food Industry Association), fmi.org/our-research/supermarket-facts.

Tracking it this way: The website for the Meat, Poultry and Egg Product Inspection Directory, provided by Food Safety and Inspection Service, USDA, is fsis.usda.gov/regulations_&_Policies/Meat_ Poultry_Egg_Inspection_Directory/index.asp.

16: By the Way, What's a Byproduct?

"I do not consider the stuff to be ground beef": Michael Moss, "Safety of Beef Processing Method Is Questioned," *New York Times*, December 30, 2009, nytimes.com/2009/12/31/us/31meat.html.

17: A Change in the Beef World

The Guardian *reported in July 2020*: Jonathan Watts, "Methane Rises to Highest Level on Record," *Guardian*, July 14, 2020, theguardian .com/environment/2020/jul/14/livestock-farming-and-fossil-fuels- could-drive-4c-global-heat-rise.

There are almost one hundred million cows: "Cattle (February 2019)," USDA National Agricultural Statistics Service, February 28, 2019, nass.usda.gov/Publications/Todays_Reports/reports/catl0219.pdf.

According to the USDA: Tom Capehart and Susan Proper, "Corn Is America's Largest Crop in 2019," USDA (blog), August 1, 2019, usda.gov/media/blog/2019/07/29/corn-americas-largest-crop-2019. In industry speak, a beef cow is technically the mother cow that gives birth to the cows that are raised for beef.

It reports the growth of biodynamic farms: "Demeter F.A.Q.'s," Demeter Association Inc., demeter-usa.org/about-demeter/demeter-faq.asp.

According to a joint study: "Lab-Grown Meat Would 'Cut Emissions and Save Energy,'" University of Oxford News & Events, June 21, 2011, ox.ac.uk/news/2011-06-21-lab-grown-meat-would-cut-emissions- and-save-energy.

Kresser cites a report obtained: Chris Kresser, "Show Notes: Debunking *The Game Changers* on *The Joe Rogan Experience*," ChrisKresser. com, November 19, 2019, chriskresser.com/wp-content/uploads/ Show-Notes-Debunking-the-Game-Changers.pdf.

18: When a Sixteen-Ounce Steak Is Not a Sixteen-Ounce Steak, and Other Lies

It is so rare that it represents: "FAQ," Kobe Beef Marketing & Distribution Promotion Association, kobe-niku.jp/en/contents/faq/index. html.

Back in 2015, approximately fifteen pounds of Kobe beef: "Exported Beef," Kobe Beef Marketing & Distribution Promotion Association, kobe-niku.jp/en/contents/exported/index.php?y=2019&page=8.

Olmsted called Kobe beef: Larry Olmsted, "Food's Biggest Scam: The Great Kobe Beef Lie," *Forbes*, April 12, 2012, forbes.com/sites/ larryolmsted/2012/04/12/foods-biggest-scam-the-great-kobe-beef-lie.

A 2016 investigation by Inside Edition: "Many Restaurants with Kobe Beef on Their Menus Are Not Actually Serving Kobe Beef," *Inside Edition*, April 29, 2016, insideedition.com/16132-many-restaurants-with-kobe-beef-on-their-menus-are-not-actually-serving-kobe-beef.

Final Thoughts

According to the United Nations Food and Agriculture Organization: Chris Arsenault, "Only 60 Years of Farming Left if Soil Degradation Continues," *Scientific American*, December 5, 2014, scientific american.com/article/only-60-years-of-farming-left-if-soil-degradation-continues.

"You can use a hammer": Bobby Gill, "It's Not the Cow, It's the How," TED.com, January 2020, ted.com/talks/bobby_gill_it_s_not_the_cow_it_s_the_how.

One test in Australia, in which freeze-dried seaweed: Research summarized in Tatiana Schlossberg, "An Unusual Snack for Cows, a Powerful Fix for Climate," *Washington Post*, November 27, 2020, washing tonpost.com/climate-solutions/2020/11/27/climate-solutions-seaweed-methane/.

Index

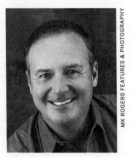

About the Author

S COTT LIVELY, president of Raise American, is an organic food entrepreneur and an absolute beef freak. Scott left a successful career in the IT industry to co-found what is now the largest organic beef company in the United States. Today, he oversees a broad portfolio of company and private labels and brands. A self-professed beef geek, he boasts that he knows every cut of beef as if he cut it himself. He divides his time between Scottsdale, Arizona, and Martha's Vineyard, Massachusetts, where he is an owner of the Martha's Vineyard Sharks, a collegiate baseball franchise that is part of the NECBL. Scott is an advocate of local economic development and regenerative farming practices applied to large agriculture.

fortheloveofbeef.com